The Poet's (40 Pound) Weight Loss Plan

Carl Nelson

Magic Bean Books

www.magicbeanbooks.co

ISBN: 9781081177836

DEDICATION

For everyone who labors through their day resigned to being overweight.

CONTENTS

CARL NELSON

ACKNOWLEDGEMENTS

"Devouring Cold Watermelon in This Anonymous River Town" was first published in CLUTCH MOV.

Illustrations are by Thawit (Tin Tin) Nelson.

Ten pages of editing were contributed by Gretchen Haupert in an effort to show me the way. All errors are mine.

"Losing weight is hard. Most diet plans will work, if people could just continue the discipline. What *The Poet's Weight Loss Plan* does differently is to conceive of weight loss in terms of the discipline required and to peel the banana from the other end. We start with the amount of discipline that the average person has shown they can sustain and design a weight loss plan from there. What most people want in a weight loss program is to continue eating as they currently eat and to lose weight as fast as is possible. *The Poet's Weight Loss Plan* is my closest approximation to this."

- the Author

Forward

"A foreword is written by someone other than the author and tells the readers why they should read the book." (- Greenleaf BookGroup). This particular forward is being written however by the book's author who has usurped the role, for two reasons. In the time that has passed since this book's publication I have changed my view of 'dieting'. That's the first. The second is that I intend to encourage you to read another book, *Ultra Processed People (The Science Behind Food That Isn't Food)* by Chris Van Tulleken. Not to worry. You may still read this one. But, since publishing this book near six year ago I have continued to gain insights into weight loss. And there are several updates I feel should be mentioned in this forward to the book.

First, though intermittent fasting has generally gained widespread popularity as a dietary strategy, a gentler time-restricted 16:8 or 14:10 mode of intermittent fasting has become quite popular. In fact, at the age of 75, I've adopted the 14:10 mode myself. A 24 hour fast as I've described in the book, plays a bit too much with my electrolytes at this stage in my life. Not only must I submit to the day of fasting, but I'm well into finishing the next day before by body feels whole again. Too much agony. But then, probably the best thing to be said of this book (aside from the fun poetry) is that it describes a healthy diet and it is an easy, lo-cost way to figure out just how much weight loss is worth to you. Do you want to spend the discipline required? You'll find out. It will become clear.

Second, of the people I know who are slender and who stay slender through their early and especially their latter years, many share a common trait. They aspire to achieve (or fight to sustain) a certain societal standing, whether within the culturally or the spiritually elite. And this requires maintaining a slender weight. It is quite amazing the sacrifices people will make to mingle among the successful. They'll literally starve day and night if they have to. If you are of this sort, chances are you are not attracted to this trailer park friendly literature. Nevertheless, here's an avenue to explore if you are trying to acquire the discipline to drop a few pounds... become a raging snob.

Finally, and most importantly, it may not be necessary that you buy this book at all. (full disclosure) I have finished reading one of the most enlightening books I have read in recent memory: *Ultra-Processed People* by Chris Van Tulleken. (Fear not. It's a bestseller! With highly credentialed sources, ample footnotes, and written by an author with several degrees from leading world institutions. Woo-who!) I encourage you to read it, if only for the incredible insights which will rock your (nutritional) world view. Here's a taste:

We have taste sensors throughout our body, even in the testes - not just within the mouth.
Cows don't just eat grass. They are incredibly sophisticated in the varieties of vegetation which they seek out and consume for their nutritional needs.
If babies are presented with many varieties of food, this will select and eat those which meet their nutritional demands. And when they have met these nutritional demands they will stop their eating.
Exercise does not burn more calories. It merely shifts where the calories are consumed - from our other tissues and organs to the muscles.
It is generally impossible for people to "lose weight" by dieting. We have a genetic disposition for fat distribution.
Fake foods are dimes on the dollar cheaper than real foods. Moreover, we can be imprinted to prefer them, and they can be flavored and textured so as to be highly addictive. For these reasons, fake foods are pushing real foods off the grocery shelves.
Supplements do not benefit us. These nutritional elements must be taken as real food.
Our natural food is incredibly complex as are our biological drives to use and select for them. The human diet of real food represents an incredibly complex web of interconnectivity.
Fake foods disrupt these bodily signals, and so have led to a plethora of chronic diseases of which a growing obesity epidemic over the past eighty years is just the most glaring.
Probably the best way to not be overweight is to eliminate processed foods from your diet. This will not only make you your natural weight, but make you feel much better both physically and mentally (with the actual re-wiring of your neural tissue).

So. There it is. Mea Culpa. But I do recommend reading this book as a good prelude to reading Van Tulleken's update. Good nutrition is important, and fasting is beneficial. You will have your dieting feet placed firmly in reality and be ready to take the next step: real food.

Plus, you'll likely enjoy the inspirational poems.

Carl Nelson
June, 2024

CARL NELSON

Preface

"Wisdom reveals the great forces at odds even over a mouse."
- Bluert Johonsen

"...or even over the weight of the mouse."
- the Author

At some point it occurred to me that people read for a reason; that is, because they want something or seek something. I had been told in my high school and undergraduate English classes that we should 'eschew transitional interests' in judging literature. That is, whether or not we enjoyed the subject, we should judge the writing independently. Good advice if you were of the mind to please critics, but for a young writer trying to find his audience, he might as well been told to stab himself repeatedly in the foot with this pen.   People generally search for what interests them first and judge the writing second... or much later than that... if ever. Good writing for most people is like the artwork on your walls and, whereas it facilitates the ambiance, goes unnoticed.

What interests people?

I entered the field of medicine because I had hoped to understand people. I imagined doctors had the tools and a prescience allowing them to virtually read my mind extending even to those parts unconscious to me. In my third year of medical school I found myself chatting away with this patient, endeavoring to plumb her soul, when all of a sudden it occurred to me - like Saint Paul looking up from the ground around his horse; *this woman wasn't here to share her soul. She was sick and wanted to be well! What had I been thinking?*

So, I drifted into the Arts.

I enjoy poems which have beauty. I enjoy poems which vivify the world around us. And I enjoy poems which create other worlds or place us in another's. I enjoy poems of philosophical maunderings. Nevertheless, I can't help but think that every poet would sigh in contentment if the value of their endeavor were measureable and not a matter of opinion - rather like a time for running the mile.   Whether or not you might like me or what I think, there it is - the winning time.

It wasn't until a year or so ago that I happened upon this successful way of becoming the weight I chose to be.   I had to tell people! Then, it occurred to me that people interested in achieving weight loss might also be interested in reading poetry about the struggle. Why not combine the two into a book of poetry and prose of obvious use? *The Poet's Weight Loss Plan* was born. I hope you enjoy the poems while becoming the weight you want to be.

A Call for Help

My breeches bloom.
My shirt blossoms.
I crunched a chair.
I cracked a settee.
Springs are busting out
all over.

A BIT ABOUT FAT

I once assisted in surgery as a medical student. My job was to hold back rolls of abdominal fat. It was surprising how thick the layer of fat on a patient could be. The body fat was a several inch thickness of yellow bubbles of fine fat globules the size of Rice Krispies, red-speckled with bleeders and slippery as all hell. Everything inside of the body is slippery, but these slabs also had the spring of shaped plumbing insulation. I struggled with the stainless steel retractors as the fat slabs would maneuver to slide from my grip with the slightest inattention and spring into the operating theater. They were a nuisance.

Even if you do not smoke or drink excessively, and otherwise live prudently, you may easily find yourself overweight. Millions do. And it's a nuisance. But it's a predilection generally assumed when you live in the affluent First World, just like Chinese take-out.

Long before I acquired Type Two Diabetes and high blood pressure I had tried to reduce my weight. Usually by our middle decades we have acquired a few more pounds than we would like and take a swing at trying some of the diet plans out there, if only for the sake of appearance. The only thing that really got the weight off was contracting hepatitis. I don't recommend it. And eventually I gained that weight back (along with my pinked up health).

By my sixties, I became even more determined to lose some weight. But with age, losing weight becomes harder. Our bodies have swollen with the gradual accretion of extra pounds. The extra fat messes with our hormones. We exercise less. We burn less fuel. We have lost muscle mass. And prepared food has gotten better and more easily available, especially as the finances and leisure time become more allowing.

In my mind, losing weight was a done deal. But each time I tried, my resolve tapered off after a couple weeks or a month. I'd lose ten pounds only to gain it back. While my body weight continued to trend upwards. What with all of the sobering statistics out there, and perverse tales in the science literature of a mind which compensated for lost weight by increasing our urge to eat - I'd about decided that my vision of the formerly slender me was unreachable, or at least, unreachable at any reasonable cost. Because I like food and am just moderately active. The insane life-style concessions it appeared a person in my situation needed to make to become and remain slender just didn't appear worth it. That is,

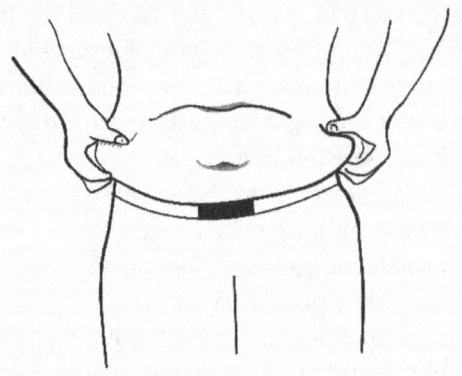

Full Disclosure

It's rather nice to be able
to grip the problem,
take a good look at it
and get a sense
of the difficulty.

until this diet, which more or less assembled itself from out of my circumstances.

Presently, (as I re-write the initial draft of this book) I have maintained this diet for 12 months and have lost 42 pounds. And better yet, I feel no hesitation about being able to continue the diet perpetually, and certainly until I reach my goal of 50 pounds weight loss. (At which point I will publish.) By internet guidelines I will still be 'obese' but inside the borderlands of overweight. But there's no need for me to stop at 50. Who knows? I might just continue until I disappear altogether. (That's a joke.) Eventually I would like to lose 65 pounds and remain at a weight of 250 pounds.

You might note that it has taken me quite a while to lose 42 pounds. But the 42 pounds is not the most important figure. What is most important is that I have kept to my plan for 12 months and am confident that I will continue. *The Poet's Weight Loss Plan is that easy to live with.*

Ode to a Donut

I smelled them from the back porch.
Completing my morning ablutions,
I hurry
through the cool morning air
to be with
the other devotees.

Fried early this morning,
fresh and squishy,
and glazed with sweet praise,

it is this floury lotus
of the bakery display case,
I bend to worship.

INTRODUCTION

Have you ever wondered why we are ruled by our emotions?
It's because reason doesn't have the chops.

Chances are this is not your first try at losing weight. Most diet plans use gentle reason to try and dissuade you from eating that donut, or a second helping of mashed potatoes, or several chocolate chip cookies. They follow your appetite around like a helicopter mother, waving diet charts, meal schedules, and lists of forbidden foods, trying to dissuade your appetite from wanting what it wants. It's rather like reasoning with a willful child. The unrepentant child (that is, your body) wants what it wants. Your inner hovering mother (which would be your self-discipline) can frazzle and tire in fairly short order.

There are oodles of diets out there, but they all have one thing in common. Few diets can manage actual sustained weight loss. Ninety-seven percent of people who lose weight gain it all back (and sometimes more) within three years, statistics say.[i] A United Kingdom study[ii] found that of those people who began new diets, two out of five quit within the first seven days. That is, a large number of us don't last at our diets much longer than a week. Only one out of five made it a month.[iii] Another study notes that "maintaining a sustained preferred weight is as challenging statistically as becoming a millionaire."[iv]

Describing good nutrition is not hard. Neither is it hard to quantify how many calories your body will burn each day, nor how many calories you are eating. What is hard is to stick to a nutritionally sound diet that will allow you to lose until you reach a specific weight and then to sustain this weight permanently. The hardest part of most diets is persistence. And a necessity of persistence is self-discipline. You must somehow always summon the self-discipline to persist.

A Successful Strategy/Playing the Odds

Most people, if they gain weight, do so quite gradually. What this all means is that by far the majority of people are successful at eating a diet that approximates their daily caloric requirements and do so without giving it a lot of thought. This is the way most people want to live. And yet the majority of people are overweight. Why?

Donut Holes

All of the stars were aligned in marketing
when they developed this brilliant evasion.
Not only are they bite-sized
so you are 'cutting back',
but there is nothing there!

Seldom do producer and ad man
so closely collaborate
in such a successful confidence game
as donut holes.
☺ ☺ ☺ ☺ ☺
I give it five smiley faces.

It's because, while slow accretion of weight is easy, losing body fat is hard and painful.

When people first try to lose weight, they generally gravitate toward diets that are simple and will dump the weight fast, so the hurt is short. Or they gravitate toward diets where the hurt is minimal, but the diets are so restrictive and complicated and the restrictions so unrelenting as to be unlivable.

Often people will be sold on a diet that requires personal change, the idea being that they must change their relationship with food. Hey, relationships are difficult! And personal change is very difficult. I've been trying to change my personality for nearly seventy years with minimal results. If you multiply the odds of changing yourself by the odds of the average person losing weight, the product is a near impossibility. *The Poet's Weight Loss Plan* is not about changing your nature; it's about limiting your nature. Every lasting success comes with limits. That's what *The Poet's Weight Loss Plan* provides.

Phantom Weight Loss

When you start a weight loss program that promises precipitous weight loss, the first ten to twenty pounds of weight loss is due largely to fluid loss. So is the decreasing waist size. When you begin eating less, your body needs to produce less saliva and less gastric and pancreatic juices for digestion. Your body normally produces six to seven quarts of these digestive juices a day. A low-calorie diet may halve this. Your body will also lose fluid as low-calorie diets typically cause a loss of electrolytes. Body fluid amounts depend upon how many electrolytes you take in, rather than the water you might drink. Added to this is the lessened weight of food in your stomach and feces (three to five times less) in your digestive tract. From ten days to two weeks out, the further loss of weight will be from your constant weight – bones, skin, muscle, internal organs and, finally, fat – the one we want to lose. This is when your precipitous weight loss plateaus.[v] This is most often when people get discouraged and quit, as they are working as hard but getting fewer results. The magic of the diet has faded.

Diets that propose gradual weight loss through better eating do not create magical gains through fluid shifts. On *The Poet's Weight Loss Plan* my weight dropped consistently about one pound per week throughout the period of about four months when I fasted one day per week. As a note, it is

'Energy' Foods

There is no such thing as 'energy' foods.
These are high calorie foods.
Go ahead,
eat a wheelbarrow full of them.
How 'energetic' do you feel?

recommended that you refrain from weighing yourself every day as your weight has natural fluctuations that can be hard on morale. I've restricted myself to weighing in once a week on the morning after fasting and before breakfast - more about weight measurement later.

Later along in my diet, I hit a plateau at around twenty-five pounds of weight loss. Thinking at first that I had increased my consumption inadvertently, I increased my fast to two days per week. My weight still did not diminish as expected. Confusion abounds when the anticipated weight loss does not occur. I suspected my scales, my eating, variations in what I wore when weighing in, variations in the time when weighing in. Eventually, after researching, I believe that I had encountered a set point plateau.[vi] These can last from one to two months and will occur when your weight loss has reached your body's current weight "set point," which can have a broad regional range of from ten to twenty pounds. This will be discussed fully in "Making Progress/In the Muddle, Right There in the Abdomen."

Yo-Yo Dieting and Metabolism

How can one person have a different metabolism than another person? I have wondered about this, and the most prominent answer is that various components of the body burn calories at various rates. For example, "Research shows that a pound of muscle burns seven to ten calories per day, while a pound of fat burns only two to three calories, according to the American Council on Exercise."[vii]. So, your resting metabolism is largely a measure of your body's composition. Your metabolism otherwise is dependent upon how active you are and other factors (gender, hormonal levels, health, etc.).[viii]

This is a clue as to why yo-yo dieting, also known as weight cycling or the repetitive gaining and losing of weight, can actually make an overweight person's situation worse. When the overweight person loses weight they lose both fat and muscle. But when they gain the weight back, they gain mostly fat. After several dietary failures, the yo-yo dieter has actually lowered their basal, or resting, metabolic rate, making weight loss even harder. This is the effect of yo-yo dieting.

A successful dietary strategy is best played out on a weekly basis and combined with exercise and good nutrition. Then the metabolic effects of backsliding (yo-yoing) are kept to a minimum.

Yo-yo dieters are reminiscent of those biblical tribes of yore who, tiring

Bite-Sized Snacks

'and why you can't eat just one'

Bite-Sized Snacks are a dieters' hazard.
They come with the territory like ticks and hunting.
Which, while you're off gunning for the larger game,
take the opportunity to hide in your clothing or hair.
If someone in the family should go out for groceries,
check them upon their return for Bite-Sized Snacks.

Once inside they will hop about the kitchen,
dining room and living room coffee table top
with the freedom of fleas.
Undetected, these snacks can cause diet failure,
weight gain, even Type 2 Diabetes.

They feign inconsequence, but they are not!
Corporations realize, for example, when you are shunning
the larger bakery items, like cherry turnovers or donuts
even when advertised as fat free or with reduced calories!
that you will buy a boxful of bite-sized jelly surprises or
powder sugared donut holes as a substitute.
What is seemingly a perfect way to 'cut back'
is *actually* a good way to expand.

of one god's strictures would try another god, then another, wandering from one deity to the next in an unrelenting search for an easier path, a more pleasurable discipline. Quick weight loss is today's Golden Calf. Weight loss is rather like being born again. But a being born-again is more apt to thrive the longer the gestation.

The Christian church, in its wisdom, has co-opted this tendency upon the part of us all to backslide, and to quit one discipline for the greener pastures of another, into the Christian week. You are given six days to wander in the wilderness. On the seventh day you are taught again. Each week is a reiteration of this wandering in the wilderness with slight variations. Over time and a long gestation, you are truly born again. You have developed a wisdom and a discipline that sticks.

Likewise, *The Poet's Weight Loss Plan*.

The Thermos Effect

Fat is a good insulator. Because of this, overweight round people tend to lose less body heat than slender long people. So round bodies compensate by running at a lower rate of metabolism in order to decrease their heat production. So round people burn fat at a slower rate than slender long people. Women also have a harder time losing weight than men because of a gender disposition for brown fat accumulation (an extra kind of fat only found in women), less muscular bodies, and the fat-accumulating influence of estrogens.

Smoking for Weight Loss

Aside from nicotine's dampening of the appetite, smoking produces weight loss by impairing the metabolic function of the lungs, heart, and liver. The smoker must take in more calories for his or her metabolism to perform at the same level as nonsmokers. If you need another reason not to smoke, there it is.

Raising Myself By My Own Bootstraps

By losing weight with *The Poet's Weight Loss Plan*,
in a small way - to date, 15 pounds -
I am literally raising myself by my own bootstraps.
How egalitarian!

One pound per week
like a yellow balloon set free
from the pull of gravity.
And there's a delight in the day
which I have manufactured.

I am creating delight now
through *The Poet's Weight Loss Plan.*
As every step becomes more genial,
more charming to myself.
I must say,
I'm being won over!

I'd never granted myself
this much esteem.
But I seem to be climbing stairs
like a returning Earl,
eager to claim his ancestral ruin.

Simplicity

You can form a simple habit. You can follow a simple plan. What is complex either won't get done or won't last because it exhausts the energies.

The Poet's Weight Loss Plan is simplicity itself: don't change what you are doing but make it even simpler by leaving stuff out. Leave out cheap carbohydrates. Leave off snack foods. Leave out candies, soda, sugar, syrups, ice cream, pastas and breads and potatoes. Many of these foods will sneak their way back in, but at a dribble, not a deluge. And they will stand out like escaped convicts in orange suits because the rules are simple: you are greatly decreasing the amount of fast-acting carbohydrates that you take in. The role of fast-acting carbohydrates will be discussed fully in "Part A: The Diabetic Type 2 Diet."

Next, leave off too-large portions. Make your diet simpler by not taking second helpings.

A lot of Americans' nutrition is adequate simply because they eat far too much. Processed foods with their empty calories wouldn't supply adequate nutrition if Americans were to eat far less. This is one reason why deciding what you eat will be important. You will need to eat foods whose calories accompany good nutrition, since you are taking in many fewer calories.

With *The Poet's Weight Loss Plan* you needn't buy differently, or prepare different meals. No need to fix one for yourself and another for the other members of the family. You keep your routine or make your routine even simpler. You eat as normal but leave out certain foods or just don't serve them to yourself. Kids might need macaroni and cheese, or French fries, or chips for energy - but you don't. You eat the chicken and vegetables. They eat the chicken, vegetables, and macaroni and cheese.

By eating less while not purchasing any specialty items required by a 'special' diet, *The Poet's Weight Loss Plan* will save you money. And when you have finally achieved your preferred weight, there is no need to transfer from some specially designed and purchased diet to your own. Your diet is already made up of the foods you normally eat and the routines you normally use. This is simplicity. Your normal household meal routine continues without a ripple. When you achieve your goal, you simply continue as you are without transition, without new habits to acquire, nothing special to buy. Rather, just a quiet congratulations.

Rebelliousness Goes to Fat Quickly

Food was life and will become life.
Wasting food is not right.
Everything about food is sacred.

Leaving food on your plate
will not make you thin.
Rather, it makes you
an undisciplined person.

Struggling against restraints
like an infant in its car seat,
is like tearing open a bag of cookies.
The whole point is *not* to eat
 just one.

Undisciplined people tend
to over-eat.
We've been through this.
Rebelliousness goes to fat
quickly.

THE POET'S WEIGHT LOSS PLAN

The Poet's Weight Loss Plan stitches two very well researched and credible dietary regimens together to produce *a diet synergy which offers you statistically your greatest chance of success.* Success means that you will meet your weight loss goal and sustain this weight permanently. This is a permanent plan. You will be reborn as the weight you choose with the discipline necessary to sustain it.

There are other benefits to this plan which we will discuss, but *the main benefit of this diet is it is nutritionally sound and produces sustained weight loss.* I am walking, breathing proof of having achieved a sustained weight of 40 pounds less than my beginning weight.

108 million U. S. citizens are currently on diets. They will make four or five attempts to diet per year. The U. S. diet industry currently boasts twenty billion dollars of revenue per year. And yet only around 3% of the citizens who currently diet will successfully sustain their weight loss. *Sustained weight loss is the holy grail of dieting.*

The Poet's Weight Loss Plan utilizes a standard Diabetes Type 2 diet regimen. This diet has been found through scientific trials by medical authorities to be nutritious and control the body's glucose levels within standard bounds when followed as described. It is safe, nutritious, inexpensive and convenient as normal eating. It's a professionally proscribed pathway which monitors your caloric intake while watching your nutrition. An added benefit is that a Diabetes Type 2 diet normalizes a person's glucose level, which prevents cyclical food gorging by dampening appetite cravings. It can also help prevent the onset of diabetes.

The Diabetes Type 2 diet will be your normal eating for six days of the week. This will be a maintenance diet. During this period of the week you will practice eating the amount of calories your body uses each day, but no more. You will feel fine. It will require no more discipline than heading off to work each day and coming home. It's just normal life. No sweat. No agony. You will look forward to meals and snacks. Unless you are currently eating way more than you need each day (and are gaining weight fast), this portion of your diet shouldn't feel much different to you than how you feel right now reading this book.

Third Pound

"Mirror, mirror, on the wall.
Who's the thinnest of them all?"
"Not you."
Not yet.

On the seventh day of the week you will fast. The fasting day is your weight loss day. Once you have attained your preferred weight, you may eliminate this day and simply treat the day as any other of the week. If, in the future, you have allowed yourself to eat a bit more than you should each day and have gained a few pounds, you evaluate and control your overeating, and re-initiate your day of fasting. It's as simple as that.

To lose weight your body must take in less calories per day than it burns, as I have stated. When this happens you will become hungry. You will not particularly enjoy this, though I will touch on some pleasures. Losing weight is not fun. If it were, many of us would die happily of hunger. No one does. Hunger is a primary drive. It will happen, and there is no way around it. It's rather like Original Sin. We're stuck with it. But, on this diet we're stuck with it for only one day a week. This is a strategically sound move.

As I've noted, 2 out of 5 people quit their diets after the first week. Only 1 out of 5 make it a month. And only 3% of those who succeed with their diets can successful sustain their weight loss.   These are the statistics. I don't have statistics for how many people can stick with their diet for one day. But I believe your chances are pretty good.

Why do I think this?

It is because *The Poet's Weight Loss Plan* stitches two of the most sought after diet desires
- eat normally
- lose weight fast

together to work synergistically. The first half of the diet is eating normally. Few of us have a problem doing this. The second half of the diet is fasting. *There is no quicker way to lose weight than by fasting.* And all of us would like to lose our extra weight as quickly as is possible. By joining these two situations we create something of a climber's chimney. By pressing his back to one side, and his feet to the other, the rock climber is able to make his way to the top of a chimney. *The Poet's Weight Loss Plan* works just like that. It takes no special skills. It takes no special meals. It is simple, but smart.

Sixth Pound

Quite hungry this morning
as I generate weight loss,
tossing energy into the void -
like a fat star diminishing itself
twinkle by twinkle.
Hostess Twinkie by Twinkie.

The 2 out of 5 persons who quit their diet after the first week had been dieting for 7 days. In this diet, you fast for only 1 day; then it's back to normal eating. It's very easy to give in after being hungry for seven days. But most of us can manage being hungry for one, especially when we rest for 6 days in between.

The Poet's Weight Loss Plan strategy is analogous to those of the great religions. As an example, Christians during the regular week try to implement and employ what they have learned during the Sabbath. During the Sabbath they take stock of where they are, are forgiven their failures and prepare themselves to start again. Whatever grace acquired over the Sabbath, they try to sustain over the following week. Just so, the real measure of the weight we lose fasting is how well we are able to sustain this loss over the following week, just as the test of Christian principles is during the week following Sunday. So our weight loss is not viable if it cannot be sustained throughout the following week. So every day is as valuable as the next or the latter. It's just that during the day of fasting we strategize so as to discipline ourselves to lose weight. Whereas during the week we discipline ourselves so as to remain the weight we are. Both hands help the other. By losing weight, we have something to sustain. And by practicing our restraint, we sustain our weight loss.

Christians know all about backsliding. It happens. But the week is only 7 days long, and on the 7th day they take stock and begin anew. So it is with *The Poet's Weight Loss Plan.* Each week we begin anew. *The Poet's Weight Loss Plan* is actually a week long diet, which begins again the next week. The specter of dietary yo-yoing is largely eliminated. Because if you fail your fast, then you miss your weight loss for that week and try again the next. You may quit the painful weight loss portion of the plan, or simply place it on pause for a period of time - without any harm - and then pick it back up again when you feel more able. *The Poet's Weight Loss Plan* is nearly as forgiving as God.

There are benefits to fasting beyond weight loss, which we will talk about in the chapter on Intermittent Fasting. There are also tricks that make a day's fast easier to manage than you might think. And there are even things to be enjoyed about fasting. We will touch on all of these later in the chapter on Intermittent Fasting.

Tenth Pound

The galaxy is fast expanding.
It seems the Universe has a waistline problem.
Too much snacking while staring into a boring void from the sofa
and thinking you can mask the gain as dark matter, I'd guess.
Existence is overweight!
God breathed across the surface of the deep
while dipping into a can of Pringles
and slurping on a Big Gulp apparently.
Poet's even, are beginning to mention the burdensomeness of it.
I pray and recommend my *Poet's Weight Loss Plan*
featuring Intermittent Fasting,
a proven path to sustained weight loss.

THE TYPE 2 DIABETES DIET

At the start of any training or effort at change there will be complaints. Benefits generally accrue at a slower pace than deprivations. It is the way of the world. Nevertheless, a Type 2 Diabetes Diet needn't put you off your feed. You can still eat everything. But the amount of carbohydrates you eat need to be balanced with the proteins and fats you feed on. And your total caloric intake cannot exceed your per diem limit.

Once you've gotten an idea how your regular eating habits stack up against this new diet, you'll be free to stitch and re-shape a new regular eating habit which suits both the diet and you. Some foods such as candies and soda pop you'll find such an egregious waste of your calories, that eliminating them altogether will be a no-brainer. Most of these will be quick acting carbohydrates which we don't necessarily love, but shovel into our mouths anyway as a very domesticated sort of addiction - quitting them gets easier as you quit eating them. Getting rid of them will be as easy as walking past them in the store. (Just say "No" to Stop & Goes.)

Responsible everyday eating can be, oddly enough, harder to accomplish than fasting. This is odd because eating responsibly is pleasant and involves no suffering from hunger pangs or cravings. It is simply a matter of staying within the guidelines, whereas fasting does involve some suffering. During a fast you will come to understand exactly how much pain is required to lose a pound. No more, no less. And you will be pleased when it's time to eat again.

The irony is that with a fast there is only one decision to be made and only one dictum to follow: no calories. You can't eat anything and that's that. It's simple, straightforward, and offers no way to rationalize one's way out. You did the crime, and now you do the time.

Fasting is easy; eating is hard. With a regulated diet, temptations and grey areas abound. It's exactly like everyday life. But if you have managed to stay out of jail, maintain relationships and are financially solvent, you surely have enough discipline and self-awareness to succeed at this diet.

Twelfth Pound

This bumper I have is a worry,
and my adversaries poke it.
Children draw me as a circle.
I pant and sweat.
I leave deep footprints.
Would you believe I've 'ballooned'?

Regularity

Regularity is an important part of eating correctly for two main reasons. The first is that regularity is easier to plan for and can become habitual. And what is habitual requires little discipline. And what requires little discipline is easy to sustain. And sustained weight loss with good nutrition is the primary goal of *The Poet's Weight Loss Plan*.
A second reason for regular meals and snacks is that we want to control hunger. And hunger is controlled by maintaining our blood glucose at a constant comfortable level. This is most closely obtained when our caloric intake is short on quick acting carbohydrates and taken at equal time intervals. (More on quick acting carbohydrates later.) When we are able to control our hunger in this way, we are better able to control our eating. Controlling our eating is essential for sustained weight loss and sound nutrition.

Portions

It's easier, the more bland the food, to watch one's portions. I rarely eat too much lettuce or celery, hog the carrots or cauliflower, or pig out on oatmeal. Snitching another greasy sausage is not above me, however. And another scoop of ice cream or a handful of potato chips is apt to get right past the port authorities. Fast acting carbohydrates and tasty delicacies create a situation ripe for corruption. It's best to refrain from purchasing any of these. If they are not in the house, they can't be eaten.

As with many things, it's the gray areas which engender the most trouble. Like lawyers, our desires race there to press for advantage. The grey area of *The Poet's Diet Plan* - and where the devil frequents - is portions. Now, if you read the Diabetes Type 2 guidelines, what comprises a portion is very clearly outlined. Nevertheless a sober, dispassionate, stern judgment is required. Initially, some work is required. And the meal docket can get backed up while weighing each spoonful, and a lot of time can get burned up in the plea bargaining and caloric accounting. Moreover each spoonful we slop onto our plate is on a 'slippery slope' fraught with temptation.

An easy way to go about this - rather than to fiddle through your cupboard for a good recipe - is to imagine the meal you would normally prepare. Then leave out the quick acting carbohydrates. And then adjust the other portions of your regularly eaten foods to fit within your *carb*

Portions
"Sufficient unto the day..."

Portion size is another grey area.
So grey, in fact,
that I'm surprised we don't see
a lot of lawyers
clustered around this poem,
haggling.

For what exactly is a portion?
Well, it's a serving.
And what is a serving?
Well, it's either tightly specified on the package side,
or you must intuit it from the recipe.
If it 'serves' six,
then one sixth of it
must be a 'serving'.

But what if you are not 'normal' size?
Surely the serving for a 120 pound woman
is not the same as for
a 300 pound man.
Oh-ho! But it is.

Portion size can be such a quagmire
of interpretation and evasion
as to puzzle the general populace.
So much so that Christ finally addressed it
in His *Sermon on the Mount*, declaring:
"Sufficient unto the day is the evil thereof."

By which, (I'm sure) He meant,
that there is no need to bother your priest in the
confessional
about your diet
 as
deep down in that hardened little gizzard of yours,
you'll know if you've taken enough.

choices (to be explained next). Take a good look. That will be the composition of your dinner the next time you prepare this meal thereafter.

Designing Your Diabetic Type 2 Diet

The following is the structure of a Diabetes Type 2 diet - which is also a healthy diet. You could do worse! (And probably are.) What you will actually eat on this diet will depend upon you: upon your food preferences, upon your love of cooking, and upon your bank account. But here are the building blocks as taken from my own lessons as a Diabetes Type 2 patient. The diet we are designing will be how you eat. It will be the foods you normally eat, and the dishes you normally cook - plus any additions or changes you would like to try. It should actually save you money as you will eat less, improve your nutrition and prepare simpler entrees.

Glucose is the common energy molecule your body creates from the food you eat. It is like a cellular currency. People with diabetes have trouble producing enough insulin to control the level of glucose in the blood. By controlling better what they eat, diabetics can regulate better the levels of glucose introduced to the bloodstream and thereby help reduce the need to produce the regulatory insulin hormone. Proper eating assists their bodies in managing their blood glucose. Chronically elevated levels of blood glucose cause problems throughout the body at a cellular level. So it is important to keep one's blood glucose within a normal range.

For people without diabetes, who can produce adequate insulin response, higher than needed levels of glucose in the blood are converted to fat. This is why eating fast releasing carbohydrates causes weight gain. Fast releasing carbohydrates produce blood sugar spikes which incite insulin release which causes fat creation. Blood sugar spikes which cause insulin spikes then cause rebound blood sugar dips, which induces a person to eat more quick sugar releasing food, which causes an insulin spike, and so on... 'Junk food' is particularly high in quick release carbohydrates - which is one reason we crave it. Some nutritionists believe the sugar high these foods produce within the brain can be as addictive as cocaine. Junk food has addictive qualities. But the less you eat, the easier it is to refuse more. A proper Diabetes Type 2 diet can also assist normal people to resist these addictive and fat producing 'junk food' fast release carbohydrates as they learn to appreciate life without the huger pang alarm system.

Thirteenth Pound

This residue of pleasure rims me
and blocks my knees
like a rising moon
offering spent wisdom
and no romance.
It is fully corpulent tonight
as it rises above the beltline.

When grocery shopping, a good rule of thumb is to buy from the peripheral walls (meats and fresh vegetables) and to shun the center aisles of the store which are flooded with quick releasing carbohydrates: quick serve foods, white breads, cereals, pastas, cookies, candies, donuts, snacks, etc..

The purpose of the Diabetes Type 2 diet is to create a normal range of blood sugar in your blood at all times through strategic eating. The core diet is built around limiting carbohydrates, and limiting portion size. This is accomplished through *carbohydrate counting*.

Carbohydrate Counting

Food is made from three types of nutrients: protein, fat and carbohydrate. Your body metabolizes these nutrients to create glucose (among many other sorts of molecules), which is the body's preferred molecule for energy. Glucose levels which are extremely high or low are hazardous to both your long and short term health, causing problems with your eyes, kidneys, nerves or heart. For your body to remain healthy and perform well, the blood glucose levels must be regulated. *Carbohydrate counting* is a form of meal supervision used by diabetics to manage their glucose levels. But it is also a handy tool for non-diabetic people to use to plan their meals in order to maintain a proper weight. (Too much glucose in the blood equals fat creation.) This is how it's done.

Carb Choices

Your meal will be built from what are referred to as *carb choices*. One carb choice equals 15 grams of carbohydrate which equals 60 calories of energy.

The term *carb choices* will also be used to quantify the various amounts of protein and fat allowed in building your meal. This is because "all aerobic organisms release stored energy through the oxidation of acetyl-CoA derived from carbohydrates, fats, and proteins" (Wikipedia). through a intracellular series of reactions commonly known as the Krebs Cycle. One molecule of acetyl-CoA is the cellular energy creation of one molecule of glucose. Protein has about the same energy density and fat

Fat Poem #4
The Wrong Crowd

Fine wine. Craft beer. Cocktails.
Oily sauces. Fragrant cheeses. Heaped plates of pasta.
Dripping, moist, succulent fat.
Ice cream. Desserts.
Flakey pastries and creamy light chocolate éclairs
with powdered or crystallized sugars
all run to fat as fast as they can.

Like Pinocchio on the isle of donkeys,
I've fallen in with the wrong crowd.

about twice the energy density of carbohydrates. But you needn't worry about any of that. *Just remember that a carb unit measures caloric equivalency.*

There are body index calculators available which will help you to figure out how many calories someone of your height, weight, age and sex uses each day to maintain their weight. Just plug in the numbers and you will get a readout. Here is one I use:

http://www.calculator.net/calorie-calculator.html

(This is a fun calculator to play about with. For example, when I was 45 years younger, I burned approximately 400 more calories/day than presently. 400 calories is about what my current exercise regimen burns per day. So, with moderate exercise I burn about what I did 45 years ago with no exercise. It seems our bodies burn about 8 calories less per day with each passing year.)

(A good question is, should I calculate my daily caloric burn using the weight I am currently, or the weight I am planning to be? This is a good question because it goes to the heart of our weight loss strategy. You should calculate your daily caloric burn based on *current* weight. This is because we want your body to be calorically satisfied during those times when you are not fasting. This both saves you discipline and trains your body to live within its caloric requirement.)

So. What to do:

1. Use one of these body index calculators to determine your daily calorie use.
    Then divide your daily caloric needs by 60 to determine the number of carb choices you should eat each day to maintain a constant weight.

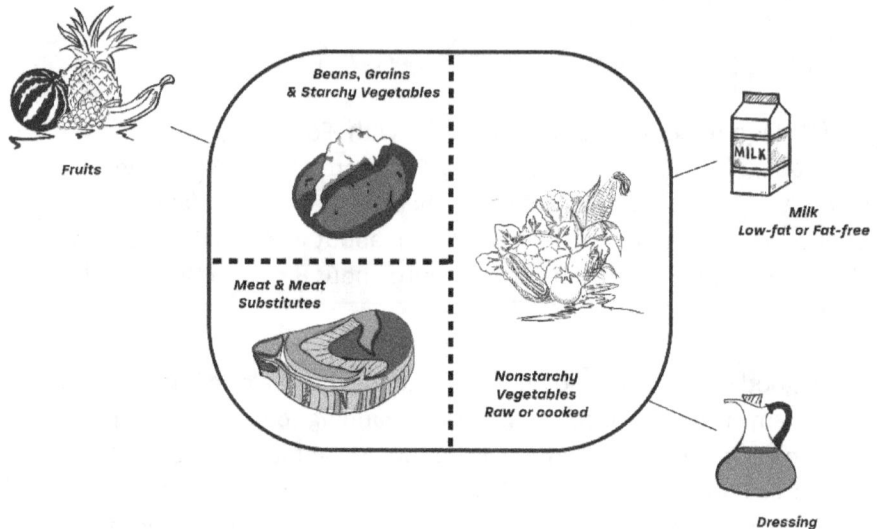

Illustration #1

The different categories of your carb choices as they should look on your plate. It's a quick, visual way to estimate correct portion size.

For example, an average male 30 years of age, 6 feet tall, who exercises 30 minutes a day, has a daily calorie burn of approximately 3000 calories.
After doing his calculations, this average male could maintain his weight while consuming 50 carb choices per day.

2. Generally, it is best to spread out our meals and intersperse them with snacks to maintain the most uniform blood glucose levels. Meals should generally be of like size, with a snack midway between each and perhaps another a couple hours after supper, perhaps as a treat with TV.

    If our normal male were to plan 2 carb choices for each of 3 snacks, this would leave him 44 carb choices to split between his 3 main meals. This would allow him almost 15 carb choices per meal.

3. Each meal is partitioned 3 ways: One quarter is your meat. One quarter are your grains, beans and starchy vegetables which comprise your quick release starches. And one half should be from your nonstarchy vegetables. (A fruit or desert would be extra carb choices, as would a caloric beverage, or a dressing.)

    So, after calculations, our normal male with approximately 15 carb choices per meal, if he were to plan his supper, could plan for 5 carb units for each of his meat and starches, 3 carb units for his nonstarchy vegetable (actually, eat as much of these as you like) leaving him the remaining 2 carb units for a beverage (such as a cup of milk) and fruit (1/2 cup) /or dessert (very sparing, probably about a bite).

    See illustration # 1.

Twenty-first Pound

If I had more money (and less weight)
I'd be eating like the wealthy
in French cooking magazines
with flapjacks nouvelle cuisine
sprinkled with bacon crumbles*
over a reduced butter/syrup concoction
and coffee freshly brewed from spring water!
It's a "lighter, more delicate dish",
made with gluten free flour
and free range egg whites.**
The syrup is sap bled from
Our Savior Jesus Trees
harvested by confirmed Catholic
native born Costa Ricans.
Presentation is emphasized.

*Vega-bacon is available on request.
**Banana slices 50 cents extra.

Meal Planning

Determining Your Carb Choices

(see APPENDIX for serving sizes of one carb choice of various items)

When you pick your carb choices you want the most bang for your buck, so your choices should be tasty, appealing, easy to prepare, nutritious and comprise a large serving which will leave you feeling full. Nonstarchy vegetables have lots of fiber and provide a lot of material to eat. 50% of your dinner plate will be nonstarchy vegetables but really, in this category the sky is the limit. Nobody ever got fat eating lettuce or broccoli or carrots or cauliflower, or green beans, etc. If you can find a way to prepare your nonstarchy vegetables in a way which makes them scrumptious, you'll be far ahead in the weight loss game. Munch non-starchy vegetables freely. You won't eat too many. (Just be watchful of what you put into the preparation.)

Starchy vegetables, grains and beans comprise one quarter of your carb choices. You might choose your starch to be the bread for your chicken sandwich. This makes lunch easy. It is very hard to get away from eating the starchy grains especially: bread, pasta, rice, potatoes. I tend to leave them out whenever convenient. For example, it's easier to cook a nice steak or chicken breast and ally it with some asparagus or broccoli topped with a bit of salad dressing or some parmesan cheese - than to bother adding mashed potatoes or some peas or corn. Pasta and rice can be tougher to eliminate or to control as so many main dishes such as casseroles and spaghettis combine them with their protein and vegetable components - and the starches usually comprise   the larger percentage component. Suffice it to say, no plan is perfect and a little adjustment can be necessary. A most important thing in these instances is to watch the portion size. (Quick starch carbs such as mashed potatoes and pastas are easy portion size violators and chronic recidivists.)

Your protein choice can be something to look forward to. If you like steak, lobster, chicken, pork, bacon, brisket, etc., then eat it. Just stay within your carb unit amount/portion size allotment.

Nutrition Facts

Serving Size 1 cup (240 mL)
Servings Per Container about 2

Amount Per Serving

Calories 230	Calories from Fat 70

	% Daily Value*
Total Fat 8g	12%
Saturated Fat 3.5g	18%
Trans Fat 0.5g	
Cholesterol 30mg	10%
Sodium 870mg	36%
Total Carbohydrate 25g	8%
Dietary Fiber 8g	32%
Sugars 11g	
Sugar Alcohol 1g	
Protein 15g	

Vitamin A 10%	•	Vitamin C 2%
Calcium 4%	•	Iron 10%

*Percent Daily Values are based on a 2,000 calorie diet. Your Daily Values may be higher or lower depending on your calorie needs.

	Calories:	2,000	2,500
Total Fat	Less than	65g	80g
Sat Fat	Less than	20g	25g
Cholesterol	Less than	300mg	300mg
Sodium	Less than	2,400mg	2,400mg
Total Carbohydrate		300g	375g
Dietary Fiber		25g	30g

Calories per gram:
Fat 9 • Carbohydrate 4 • Protein 4

Figure #2

You can check how many carb units there are per serving by checking the Nutrition Facts label on prepared foods.   A Total Carbohydrate of 15g/serving would equal one carb unit. So, in the label above for example, nearly 2 carb units (30g) is contained per serving. So in this,case eating 3/5 cup of this food would comprise one carb unit.

Fats, Dressings and Sauces

Fats, dressings and sauces are very high calorie items, so they should be used in moderation. Look up how many calories in a tablespoon of some of your favorites and keep this in mind when "adding for taste". The good news is that fat choices have slow carb release, so that they will quell your hunger for a good length of time without the rebound of quick releasing starches or sugars. So, for example, cheese (eaten in moderation) can be a real friend here. Some cheese can be a great snack, killing your hunger until the next meal. Or, if you're on the go and a scheduled meal has to be put off, a chunk of cheese is easy to eat and fairly easy to come by. Plus, it's nutritious. That fat in your steak and beef will help hold you for some time. Moreover, fat brings out the flavor in foods. So being able to rely on dressings and sauces and butter can greatly enhance your disciplined eating experience. The more you enjoy your eating, the easier time you will have maintaining your dietary habits. This is all good.

What to Drink

Water and/or plain coffee and tea are the easiest and most calorie free ways of hydrating. But one cup of whole milk is about 150 calories, half of which come from fat which make it not only nutritious, but a good snack which releases its glucose slowly. If you like milk, drink it. Just don't forget to add in the calories.

A light beer is about 100 calories a 12 oz. bottle. A glass of wine is around 125 calories for a 5 oz. serving. Alcohol can actually cause a lowering of your blood glucose, so a frosty beer plus a glass of water with my meal is an attractive dinner choice. Coffee or tea is my breakfast choice. And otherwise and at all times it's water. Water is prevalent; it's filling; it has no calories and actually helps flush calories. Drink it. Have a glass of water handy wherever you're sitting, so that it's there when you feel like reaching for something to eat. It will help. If plain old water is just too plain, and/or you feel the need to spend money, buy sparkling water or add a lemon or lime.

Soda pops and sugary/fruity drinks come with a lot of quick releasing sugars *and* calories. They are always *off* the eating list. They are a poor way

Twenty-ninth Pound

There's a lot of spent pleasures,
cheap thrills and festivities
resting in that load of triglycerides, free fatty acids,
phosphatides, sterols
and other of the low life building blocks
left outside and dumped around my middle,
like old ice chests, cars on blocks,
rusted BBQs and busted recliners.

to hydrate and a worse way to get nutrition. Eating quick releasing sugar for hunger is like drinking seawater for thirst. The rebound will be worse than the initial pang. There are much better ways to spend your calorie allotment. And avoid diet drinks with artificial sweeteners. Studies associate them with weight gain and sugar cravings.

Diabetes Type 2 Recipes

There are also lots of Diabetes Type 2 recipes available at websites sites such as this: http://www.diabetes.org/food-and-fitness/food/what-can-i-eat/food-tips/quick-meal-ideas/

Snacks

You'll need to eat some. Meals will last you about 4 hours, but are spaced about 6 hours apart.

Do not do what's easy and reach for that bag of chips, crackers, a donut, muffin or pastry. Something with a slow release sugar and/or some fat is a better choice. My favorite snacks are an apple with cheese, or a banana, a bite or two of a saved pork chop or a chicken wing, a ham slice wrapped around some cheese, some cauliflower with ranch dressing, or simply a few forkfuls of yesterday's dinner leftovers. Be a healthy seagull, but don't browse. Eat your snack and quit. Then polish it off with a big glass of water. Enjoy the swell.

Try to keep chips and candy, cakes, muffins and pies far away from your mouth and preferably out of the house.

Dining Out

Please don't be one of those people who take their dietary needs out on a waiter, friends and relations. Especially gratuitously, such as the shticks we've seen these impossible characters perform in film comedies. The reason menus advertise offered items is because that is what is offered. And your friends and relations may not want to hear

.

Thirtieth Pound

I'm just a wick
coated with surfeit,
"huff-puff"ing in the gym
burning my candle
at both ends
to consume the tallow
in the middle.

that you can wear a 32 waist size, or that your diet has been a success. Keep it to yourself. Maybe keep that light under a bushel ...please.

That said, you do need to take control of the experience, especially if dining out is a major amount of how you eat. It's best, of course, to not eat out. Eat at home. Prepare your own food. Buy your own food. This keeps it simple, will save you money and possibly time.

But, if you do need to eat out, the first thing to do is to plan for it. If you're heading into a restaurant where it is hard to control the portion size, allow yourself some wiggle room. For example, you might try eating a late breakfast and trading lunch for a late afternoon snack so that you arrive at the restaurant with some carb choices to burn and a calm appetite.

I dislike wasting food and moreover, if food is there, I tend to eat it. Table breads and chips are real hazards. Appetizers are simply an invitation to overeat. Don't order the appetizer and try to keep the chips and bread to the far end of the table. A good rule for not overeating is to keep the food out of reach. If you can't reach it, you can't eat it. So here are a couple ideas. Sit at the far end of the table. Don't ask anyone to pass you any food. Say, "No", when asked if you want some. A way I do this is to order a large light beer and to concentrate upon it. Beer is easy to concentrate on. I do it all the time.

`   Or have a coffee.

Never to order the buffet. Skip the dessert. Take a forkful of someone else's if pressed. Ordering a big salad is a good way to stay in there with the meal eaters, but not to wolf down a large portion of calories. This is why restaurants offer them. Unfortunately, they also mark you as a 'dieter' - which is kind of a buzz kill. Another technique is to survey the menu looking for choices which offer extreme savor in lieu of bulk. Say, for example, a palm sized fillet mignon drizzled with a special sauce aside some fresh asparagus. Go for those, and drink water (or a beer, or a glass of wine). People will admire your discrimination. They might even think you have culinary cred.

I doubt very much that this is your first diet attempt, so you may have a 'skill set' for these events which would dwarf mine. What we've discovered ourselves is always our most valued knowledge. And when we've earned it, we use it. It's all good. But, as a parting gift, I would send you to this link, which offers a carb choice listing of offerings at many of the favorite dining franchises in the USA. Take a look. Carb choices aren't hard to master. And in a short while you'll be estimating and slapping together

CARL NELSON

"Explode Into Space"

Loving your fat
is letting it go.

Energy equals mass times waistline squared.
You're sitting on a nova.
Set it free.

"I love smoke and lightning."
"...explode into space!"

your next meal order like a (sustained and slender) veteran.

"Nutrition in the Fast Lane" by Lily USA
http://www.fastfoodfacts.com/

Parting Pep Talk

It might seem odd, but keeping to the 'eating' portion of your diet - even though it will meet all of your needs for variety, taste, and amount - will be harder than the fasting portion. This is because for the fasting portion of the diet all you have to do is say, "No". Then you just watch the time pass (or not) while your fat is quietly eliminated. The eating portion of the diet will naturally demand a lot of negotiations with the food that's available. The ways to sin are innumerable. Here again, the diet borrows from religion. It's fairly easy to behave on Sunday morning. It's the rest of the week where the temptations flower. (Especially those weekend football games.) Each Sunday we learn how to handle the rest of the week. And the rest of the week we practice. Likewise with *The Poet's Weight Loss Plan*. Mastering the fast will lose that weight for you. But mastering the eating portion of the Plan is what will sustain that slender you, which you worked so hard for. Remember, statistically, your odds of success are very good. 80% of people generally maintain the weight they are. All you need to do is to lower the weight you are maintaining.

To master this diet, you must utilize each portion of the diet to encourage and to motivate the other. When you are fasting, imagine the pound of fat you are losing. Remember this pound of fat when you start to eat again and how proud you are to have it gone. Use this to maintain your poise and discipline. And when you eat, think of yourself as a more slender person. Feel how much easier it is to stoop and bend. Recall the lightness and flexibility that came with fasting. Do you want to let what you have worked so hard to achieve drift away?

Again, *The Poet's Weight Loss Plan* diet strategy is like the rock climber's strategy who braces his back and feet against opposite walls in order to climb the smooth chimney. It looks impossible, and it would be - except for the guy/gal with a winning strategy.

Decreasing My Existence

If the world weighs heavily on you,
you might try fasting -
decreasing your existence
until the burden feels about right.

INTERMITTENT FASTING / RUNNING ON EMPTY

Fasting has a long history and is an important component of many traditions. For Charismatic Christians, Google notes: "Fasting is done in order to seek a closer intimacy with God, as well as an act of petition." Fasting has also been used in many (sometime sketchy) health schemes as a way of 'cleansing the body'. Professional fasters in the 19th century, such as Succi and Merlatti, two Italian exhibition fasters, staged fasting 'exhibitions' or 'stunt fasts' to which they sold tickets in order to raise money. In 1885 Merlatti fasted in Paris for 50 days.

The point here is that there is nothing new about going without food for various lengths of time. In our evolution it was no doubt quite common for our ancestors to find themselves without something to eat for days at a time, or just to miss a meal or two. Fasting is an experience humans have evolved with.

If you have a health problem which might be exacerbated by fasting, or a condition which would cause fasting to harm you, you should certainly talk to your doctor before attempting the fast. If you have diabetes, high blood pressure, or are pregnant especially, a consultation with your doctor beforehand should occur. There are various levels of diabetes, and a fast which doesn't bother me, might be dangerous for you to attempt. Aside from these conditions (plus, note the *'Concerns'* following), most people can go without food for a day without incurring a health problem. They just get hungry.

Your body will not lose weight without objections. We all know what it feels like to be hungry. We all know how delicious food can be. Weight loss will be painful. Some diets would have you spread your caloric restrictions out and to specifically target foods to eat which are low in calories but high in bulk so as to make you feel as full as possible and as little hunger as is possible. These diets are strategized as if it were the *amount* of hunger which make persons quit their diet plan. I believe statistics show this to be false. The problem is that these strategies call for a person to make *continual* decisions as to what and when and how much they should be eating, and to endure *chronic* caloric deprivation i.e. hunger.

Too many decisions use up discipline. And chronic hunger saps discipline. This is why I believe the these diet plans fail us.

Fasting

Fasting is exactly how hard it is to lose weight.
No more, no less.
It is rare in life to get exactly
what you pay for.
Just this, in itself
ought to recommend it.

Pleasant or not,
just getting a fair deal in this life
is worth exploring.
And from there,
who knows what bounty might unfold.

The Poet's Weight Loss Plan believes in biting the bullet. We think dieting should be a little like removing a band aid. Best to just rip it off! Be comfortable throughout the week. And on the day you decide to lose weight, do just that. Nothing else. The decision is simple. You eat no calories for a 24 hour period. No decisions need be made. No special diet need be arranged. There will be the pain of hunger, but you have already made up your mind about that. The other days of the week you will work at generating the habitual eating habits which sustain the weight loss you will achieve on the seventh. There is nothing like a little pain to make a person feel like they are achieving. In this way, both sides of the diet create some rest from the other. On the one hand we have a comfortable life and on the other, maximal achievement! There is no faster way to lose weight than by fasting (unless you would be an extreme athlete).

And now, *The Poet's Weight Loss Plan* will offer you some tips for finding your way through a day's fast with the least pain possible.

Tricks to Fasting

My first (and last) advice is always *simplicity*. To make the fast simple, make it absolute. No calories. You may drink water or black coffee, or tea or any other naturally calorie free beverage. (Remember: avoid diet drinks and artificial sweeteners.) This does two things. First it makes the decision process straightforward and, in fact, unnecessary. Second, coffee and tea contain stimulants which also assist in raising your basic metabolic rate. If you already drink coffee, continuing protects you from withdrawal symptoms. And water allows you something to imbibe while filling your stomach. Water provides a stomach volume which is reassuring .

Simplicity is important because a hungry mind is like a child. A hungry mind will come up with whatever rationale there is that gets it fed. And fending off these distractions which create the need for special decisions and allows for special circumstances destroys discipline by chewing up the mental energies and creating loopholes you'll soon be driving donut trucks through! It is like removing your thumb from the hole in a dam. Don't do it! That's what the fables tell us.

The rule of *simplicity* also suggests fasting regularly on the same day each week. This is a good way to form a habit. And what we do

Dinner, Pass Me By

Fasting persons are like the dead.
We drift about topically.
We ghost meals.
We used to speak with food in our mouths.
Now we are too peculiar.
Since to visit and not eat is rude,
fasting people generally feel that it is best
not to show, altogether.

habitually, no longer takes discipline. Plus, your fast can be anticipated and planned around - both by yourself and others.

One of the first things you will notice when fasting is the amount of time in your day fasting will free up. If you consider the time spent planning, purchasing and preparing food, and then add the time spent dining - it may come to around *six hours of extra time*. So it is best to have some ideas ready. Otherwise, you might panic when surveying these extra seven hours without food.

A good idea right off the bat is to look at this free time as a blessing. (Which is a good way to look at everything.) You are getting a quarter of a day off. What would you like to do? Here are some ideas.

Read in the morning through your breakfast coffee, or sit outside and listen to the birds wake up. How often do we have the opportunity to do this?

Work through lunch, or take a walk. You'll either get more done, or the exercise will decrease the hunger pangs. Exercise is a proven hunger killer.

Your regular dinner time is a great time to visit the gym. The equipment and pool will be less crowded and the exercise will not only burn off more calories, but it will kill your hunger for some time afterwards. I find when I swim on the day I fast, I actually feel better in the water.

When you get home, get involved in a good book or watch a movie. Go to bed early. Think about the fine breakfast you will have in the morning.

The worst day of fasting is the first. And the worst part of the first is usually early afternoon. Drink water. Stay out of the kitchen or snack area. Don't walk into any Quick Stops now - or ever. They have nothing you need. Have something to do, or take a nap. Stay busy. But sleeping through your fast is also fair play.

Wake up the next day well rested, and find yourself not much hungrier than any other morning. Fix yourself a favorite meal, but within the guidelines

After some months spent fasting, you may find that a smaller portion fills you up. As I continued to fast and was in the fifth month of *The Poet's Weight Loss Plan,* I noticed that I could not eat as large a portion of food, such as we will when working our way down the birthday buffet, for

I Miss My Craziness

Something happened with my urge to eat.
It's become ho hum.
I look forward to lunch
more or less as a break in the day.
I miss those days as a lo-life,
mounding up the whipped cream on that wedge of pie
and the greedy urge to over-indulge.
Nowadays, more and more, it just seems stupid.

Once you can stop,
being addicted isn't fun.
The diet book just sets there, un-heeded.
The refrigerator is just another appliance.
I don't chew much,
but still drink a little,
while watching TV,
and surf for another crazy compulsion.

example, without a stomach ache.I also noticed that on the evening of my fast's second day the food around me was very tempting as was usual. But after waking in the morning and eating a normal sized breakfast, food had lost its glamour. A sugary donut was not as compelling. I didn't need any more. I didn't need a snack. After several months on this diet, I felt my romance with food had matured. We still loved each other but take the time to go off and do other things.

As an odd note: You might think that a person committed to a fast would stay out of the kitchen. And I do stay away from cooking. But I noticed this during a particularly rough afternoon without food. I was seated in the kitchen area while my wife was preparing a 'wedding soup' with Italian meatballs and pearl pasta for her and my son. The aroma was intoxicating. And I received a lot of pleasure from it! No calories were imbibed. And I felt more relaxed and more at ease seated there sniffing it all in. And the evening went easier afterwards. Certainly a lot of pleasure from eating arrives in the smells. Could it be that delicious smelling food can take some of the edge off of our hunger, and add to a diminished pleasure - rather than to irritate?

And finally...

Don't make a big deal of either fasting or your diet. Any conversation you have with others regarding your fast will only make it a larger item in your eyes. It is no big deal. You just didn't eat for a day. Nothing here to print above the fold. Let your trim body speak for itself; they'll notice.

Fat Poem #2

They either see your stomach coming
or your rear going.
Everyone knows it's the first and last things said
which lodge in the memory,
form that first impression,
into which the remainder of all that I say will be poured
and set the narrative.

My fat has gone rogue.
"No. This is not me," I would object.
But they are already staring
and snarking:
"Invasion of the Body Snatchers!"

I have emotions! I have feelings!
I have come up with some good solutions
to the problems we discussed!
But they don't see it.

OTHER BENEFITS OF FASTING BEYOND WEIGHT LOSS

Convert that useless flab around your midsection into quick cash!

Right off the bat and without doubt, fasting will save you money. That's right. I estimate that I save around $25 in meals for each day I fast. When I fast 2 days/week, this equals $50/week in food savings. Over the month this calculates out to over $200/month saved! ("Hey, we can turn on the furnace now, honey!") And, if you're like me and like to add the saved sales tax, that would make it about $220/month. Add to this the amount I would have to make in untaxed pre-income to generate this chunk, and we come up with having to earn an appreciable income of more than $300/month. to equal the amount of money saved by fasting 2 days/week. (Now, you're thinking, "That's real money! A car payment or better. Maybe I talk my significant other into it and we save $600/month.") And if we calculated in the time, trouble and expense of creating those meals, and then add to this the amount of time in earnings it would take you to save $600/month...?!

You might think of it this way. For a man the age and size of myself, each day I fast eliminates a pound of fat. Which means each pound of fat I am carrying around is worth $25. How many of us wouldn't like to cash out a few pounds of fat?

If you are currently 100 pounds overweight, you are walking about carrying a money belt worth $2500.

Reduces Inflammation

I noticed about six months after beginning my diet that I had not been bothered either by the arthritis in the index finger of my left hand, nor with the synovial cyst enlargement of my right wrist. Granted the symptoms of these come and go historically. But the symptoms had been present before, and they have disappeared for the past year.

Science indicates that fasting can assist in reducing inflammation. And after the disappearance of my own arthritic symptoms, I wondered if perhaps fasting had any effect upon autoimmune diseases. Well, there are scientists who suspect that fasting can have a curative effect on autoimmune diseases such as lupus, multiple sclerosis, et al. Clinical

Fat Poem #3

Unexciting.
Dormant fat.
Winter snows recede.
The quail sings.

Time to place it
back in the refrigerator,
back in the cupboard,
back in the flour and sugar bin,
bag it up and take it
back to the store.
Take it off your bill.

trials on mice and limited trials on humans found a significant reversal of the symptoms of multiple sclerosis. Experts caution however that these results are very preliminary. Anecdotal evidence does exist however. Moreover, there is some learned opinion that it is inflammation rather than cholesterol levels which predispose to cardiovascular disease. Reducing inflammation is a big health plus.

Youthfulness

It is hypothesized that the 'oxidative damage' to cells which occurs normally is reversed by fasting which causes the cells to cannibalize broken and aged lipids, protein and DNA. It is conjectured that, early in our evolution, periods of fasting occurred naturally during times of food shortage, and that the body put these shortages to good use in 'housekeeping activities'. Our regular modern diet eliminated these 'spring cleanings' it is thought and made us more vulnerable to the effects of aging.

In older women, there appears to be a connection between fasting and greater egg viability and fertility, that is, if we are to generalize from mice.

Professor Longo of the University of California Longevity Institute has shown that fasting for as few as three days can entirely regenerate the immune system. It is also believed by others that fasting can decrease skin wrinkles, increase cellular health, extend our lives plus perk up the immune system. Fasting has also been shown capable of reversing Diabetes Type 2 illness. It has also been shown to decrease inflammation and "theoretically may help protect the brain". In fact some research suggests that fasting and exercise work through similar pathways to cannibalize broken and junked cellular structures during the glucose shortage, while the brain grows additional neurons.

Fights Declining Testosterone Levels

Not only does losing fat help prevent diabetes, but it *helps fight the declining testosterone levels which occur with age*. Fat plays a part in changing your androgens into estrogens. That tire around your midline is feminizing you.

Ulysses, *A Poet's Weight Loss Plan* Exemplar

Apparently our fatty tissue
converts our circulating androgens
into estrogens, fellas.
That tire around your midsection
is pimping you out.
It's making you somebody's bitch.

That demand for another beer
is becoming a whine, my friend.
Your pecs are enlarging, sagging,
starting to swing!
You're on the chocolate donut with pink sprinkles path
to gender dysphoria.

You know the story about brave, manly Ulysses,
whose crew went ashore and finding a strange enchantress
were fed and feted lavishly,
and transformed into pigs?
"Squeal like a pig! Who's your daddy now?" cried Circe.

But Ulysses, who eschewed carbs
and practiced intermittent fasting,
not only was *not* turned into a muck-sucker,
but made Circe his lover, *who*,
after a year's pleasure,
packed him a lunch
and gave him directions back to his wife.

Be like Ulysses!

There are a number of the subtle things I have noticed after losing 40 pounds. I have become slightly more assertive. My desires seem more prone to express themselves. And I am less apt to scan for relationship levels when conversing; I say more what I think, and read less into their reaction. It's nice.

Stomach 'Shrinkage'

Since beginning my two day fasting periods, my stomach feels to have shrunk. A large helping, which used to fill me up, now makes my stomach ache. It has become painful to overeat, as I have done in the past with birthday parties, and celebrations of all. I feel stuffed, much earlier in the process.

Studies indicate that we do not decrease the resting size of our stomachs (which is around 0.2 liters) through fasting. Rather fasting reduces the *distensibility* of our stomachs. For example the maximum "gastric accommodation" of a human stomach is around one liter. Fasting can reduce this *distensibility* by a third or more.

Fasting Gets Easier

One of the big benefits of fasting for weight loss is that you know the effort is directly eliminating your body fat. You are wasting no time. You can't lose fat any faster than fasting except by adding exercise. One day equals so many calories, which equals so much fat eliminated. Each hunger pang is the disappearance of another little bubbly yellow mouthful of your body fat.

You can even calculate how many days of fasting to reach your goal - which will happen if you keep to your regular weekly Diabetes Type 2 diet. Use the formula: Pounds to lose/ Pounds lost per fasting day = Number of weeks till goal is achieved.

For example: I want to lose 50 pounds. I fast one day per week and I lose one pound of fat per day fasted. 50/1 = 50 weeks to achieve my goal.

I once attended a one-person theatrical about a fellow who, with

Prana for Lunch
(fasting, day two)

I believe I could live on air.
Wouldn't want to,
but this isn't bad.
No folderol around breakfast.
Just a nip of black coffee, if you please.

If it weren't for something inside
tapping its finger,
hungry and grumbling... soon to be pacing.
A thing which is not me, to my surprise,
but some relentless other

from which my fast detaches me,
to float above the ox cart, transcendent,
flitting from the ox's ear to the master's whip,
and bouncing three hops ahead of the hungry dog
to find my next crumb, my next worm, my next seed.

Do mystics fast to leave their flesh?
Is this how the soul is freed?

his parents and their friends, constituted The Pickle Family Circus. He demonstrated learning to perform a hat trick which involved rolling the hat by its brim down an arm and across his back from one hand to the other. Every week as he continued the attempt, his father would stop briefly to assess his progress and say, "more practice". Finally, the boy accomplished something which appears so difficult as to be magical.

Practice and repetition are the tools humans are given in order to perform 'miracles'. And it seems to work for everything, even fasting. Whether it is because I am more accustomed, as the year has passed, or be it simply a matter of practice - who can say how repetition works its miracles - but fasting has become easier.

...and Easier

Years ago when I initially tried fasting, I fasted once a month. And going without food for a day was tough. Since I began *The Poet's Weight Loss Plan* many months ago, I have gone from fasting one day/week to fasting two days/week and the fasting has gotten easier. My two day fast is more and more becoming an expanse of free time and less and less a source of suffering. My body seems to have gotten better at switching from burning glucose to burning fat (ketosis). The transition, which feels to occur early afternoon of the first day, has been tamed. My hunger is there, but resting quietly like my dog nearby. I have a routine to fill the time and no longer dread the advent of my fast, but choose to look forward to the opportunity to lose weight rapidly and enjoy the added free time.

The Poet's Weight Loss Plan Comes With Motivational Poetry

Fasting and dieting are natural multi-taskers
which not only leave room for other endeavors
but, in fact, clear the table.
Find yourself at loose ends?
I might be because fasting
not only cuts the fat,
it cuts the shopping,
handles the cooking
and voids the dishes.

You can diet while you swim,
make love,
go for a walk,
sit and think,
read, knit, play cards, play scrabble,
ride a bicycle,
drive to work,
put in a day's work,
enjoy the woods, beach, shopping, friends,
read a magazine,
pet the dog,
sleep.

Losing weight is an achievement
which takes care of itself,
toots its own horn,
is universally respected,
leads to better health
and pole vaults you right up there into that exclusive community
 - where people are so proud
they walk around in their bathing suits!
While the other more billowy dressed beseech them,
"How did you *do* that?"

Tell them,
The Poet's Weight Loss Plan.

Fasting's Spiritual Side

*"**Inedia** (Latin for "_fasting_") or **breatharianism** /brɛθ'ɛəriənɪzəm/ is the belief that it is possible for a person to live without consuming _food_. Breatharians claim that food, and in some cases _water_, are not necessary for survival, and that humans can be sustained solely by _prana_, the vital life force in _Hinduism_. According to _Ayurveda_, _sunlight_ is one of the main sources of prana, and some practitioners believe that it is possible for a person to survive on sunlight alone. The terms breatharianism or inedia may also refer to this philosophy when it is practiced as a _lifestyle_ in place of the usual _diet_."*

- Wikipedia

Do not practice Breatharianism. People who do not eat food and drink water die. "There are more things in heaven and earth, Horatio, than are dreamt of in your philosophy," sayeth the Bard - but death from thirst is pretty certain.

On the other hand, my experience during day two of fasting gives insight into how some mystics might have become Breatharians. And my fasting has revealed possibilities as to why mystics throughout time have fasted as a practice.

On the second day of fasting, the pressing pangs of hunger which appear about midway through the first day's fast are dulled and feel... 'remote'. The mind feels clearer, the body lighter, while the hunger is detained somewhere within as a vague impatience. It's as if hunger has become a beast confined to a basement room whose nervous shuffling and pacing one vaguely feels, but which isn't a part of you. It's as if hunger has taken with it many of your bodily needs and separated them from your mind which seems to rise lighter and clearer... 'unencumbered', almost like a soul. My guess would be that it is this 'freeing of the soul' which mystics find so useful with fasting. My materialist side would suggest that what happens during a fast is that our bodily cognition is pulled, or oriented strongly by our starving autonomic nervous system, leaving our higher mental centers to feel more 'detached'.

Whatever the mechanism, the value of this phenomena to *The Poet's Weight Loss Plan* is in producing an intriguing mental state which can be both investigated and enjoyed. We are offered the opportunity to do more

Fasting / Taken 2 the Limit

To fast,
you don't eat.
Until eventually,
what you don't do
can seem reasonable.

You adjust,
your belt, for example.
Your dinnertimes.
Your thoughts.

Beauty becomes more and more
prominent,
and food the stuff of dreams..
Your thoughts float like balloons as
eventually they put you in the corner,
where you're no trouble, either.

No meals. No bowel movements.
A little gas passes.
That's all.
You are intensely disciplined
like the lotus.

than just suffer for lack of food during our fasting. We are also, given the opportunity to investigate a previously unexperienced mental state with many pleasant qualities. For one example, my daily swim goes much better when fasting.

Why not make the most of this, if it helps us to lose weight?

Whenever a person is trying something hard, it is useful to make a list of the good things the suffering will provide. Fasting burns calories, and also allows us to better examine what might be thought of as the 'spirit'. Some spiritual examination is always good. And it's a good idea to keep these matters of the spirit in mind. They will help you to maintain a positive mindset. And a positive mindset requires much less discipline than a negative mindset. And this means that you are much more likely to persist in your endeavor. And this accomplishes *The Poet's Weight Loss Plan's* first priority. We don't quit.

...Further Spiritual Guidance

Beware of Goals / Beware of Focusing

As they say, if you are a hammer, the entire world looks like a nail. The nature of a hammer is to focus. And the point of the focus is to hammer the nail: its goal.

In a like manner, focusing on a diet, is to focus on eating, and whether we are focused on eating less or more, the nature of the focus is to think about food more even when the point is to eat less. We obsess about this meal, or the lack of this meal. If all you think about is food, this is where you are bound to end up.

This is why part A of *The Poet's Weight Loss Diet* is to eat *normally*. The less we need to think about the details of eating, the less discipline is required to sustain the diet. Any person only has so much discipline; some more than others. But a good strategy doesn't allow you to exhaust the discipline which you possess by frittering it away on complexity and slavish perseverance.

A narrative has focus. It is a natural eater. You must eat one event after another to create a narrative. This is because a narrative has a point and a goal. Like a shark, it gobbles. A narrative naturally develops into a big fat story, because eating is its character.

Swimming with Hunger

during a fast
is like sliding your arms up through a silk blouse,
swinging them trim and slender,
under and over
to stride the lane as a top model.

Fasting is an opening blossom
in a garden just prior to Eden
and a feeling so Zen - without all that clapping,
and so effortful in effortlessness,
so devoid of itself,
as if swimming off into pure absence.

Advanced Awareness

A poem, on the other hand, does not need to proceed, does not need to get anywhere, and simply describes being. So a poem does not eat and is rather like a fast. A poem does not eat because it does not try to get anywhere. A poem simply is. A poem describes being.

In fasting terms, a poem is a Breatharian. It lives on air and light. A poem can be large or small depending upon how large or small *it* is. A narrative, on the other hand, will be large or small, depending upon the events it has eaten, or is planning to eat, when it finds the fridge.

Poetry is much like fasting. And about as many people like poetry as enjoy fasting. Most of us enjoy eating, even Poet's ironically. Most of us enjoy a good story. It is healthy to eat and to listen to good stories.

But when we eat with a poetic mindset, we are not eating to fill a narrative, and the necessity of eating will not become cumulative. And having eaten this, we will not necessarily have to eat that. Poetry can assist with this. In fact, while eliminating food from the narrative tyranny, we might also consider what other desires we might consider poetically.

Thirty-fourth Pound

I'm becoming mystical about your absence,
as your matter becomes energy.
$E = MC^2$
Also paranoid
as The Laws of the Conservation of Energy
and Mulder predict:
"The fat is out there."

FULL DISCLOSURE

Diarrhea and Fainting (Hypotension)

When an individual does not eat and drinks only water, they not only do not take on calories and nutrients - they also continue to lose electrolytes through their bowel and other secretions. If you do not replace the electrolytes which are lost and not replaced with meals, then you will lose blood volume. Blood volume is not determined by the amount of water you drink, but by the amount of electrolytes you take in. Low electrolytes can create low blood volume, which can make a person *hypotensive* (low blood pressure).

Hypotensive episodes can occur especially when rising from a sitting posture, or when walking, or after eating, or relaxing in a hot tub following exercise if you have some electrolyte deficiency. These episodes can manifest by *fainting* and falls. And falls due to loss of consciousness can cause severe injury. (Imagine fainting at the top of some stairs, or into a hot tub or pool.)

Drinking water while fasting without supplemental electrolytes will make a person's blood *hyposmotic* (less electrolytes/volume) to normal blood osmolarity. Blood low in electrolytes can be dangerous because of the heart's need for electrolyte consistency, to prevent arrhythmias. Moreover, hyposmotic blood can cause the empty bowel - when *hyperosmotic* food is first introduced after fasting - to suck water from the body and into the digestive tube causing severe diarrhea.

Moreover, for the diabetic, hypotensive episodes can be confused with a *hypoglycemic* (low blood sugar) episode - though the symptoms are somewhat different.

I've found that hypotensive episodes can be most frequent the afternoon *after* breaking my fast, rather than during. I conjecture this is because of the extra blood volume used by my intestines for digestion.

For these reasons, replacement electrolytes should be taken when fasting. Normal sports electrolyte replacement drinks such as Gatorade are not recommended. This is because they also supply calories in the form of quick acting sugars which is something we are trying not to imbibe. Once the fasting body has cycled into ketosis, we do not want to lose those gains by supplying more easy to use glucose. For this reason I began taking Volt capsules by Toniiq. They contain sea salts. I preferred the capsules, as

Solving the Metaphysical Problem of the Donut

Turning it in my hand,
presents a conundrum
as it's delicious in every direction.

Tracing this mandala of empty calories,
like a swan circling a pond
glazed by the sweet sun
around a central vacancy
with my sticky finger,
while sipping coffee...

it's fabulous in every parameter I've measured.
And though its paranormal abilities have yet to be documented,
it *can* enter and leave my dreams.

drinking sea salts mixed with water is distasteful and can induce nausea.

Unfortunately, my doctor found that my uric acid levels were too high. She thought it might be a side effect of the diuretic I take for my high blood pressure. But I was also suspicious of the sea salts. My internet research indicated sea salts could increase one's uric acid levels. Because of this I switched to "Saltstick caps", an electrolyte capsule whose composition of salts is clearly measured and specified.

I've found that the solidity of my post-fast stools are a practical indicator or how well I am maintaining my fasting electrolyte levels. Taking one capsule in replacement for each lost meal gives me good stool results. You will have to experiment to find the right replacement amount for yourself. Note that I am about twice the size of a usual person (6'8", 300 pounds)

On another note: Our stools are initially yellow in color, then become brown as they are worked on by the microbes as they make their way down our digestive tracts. If you develop diarrhea immediately after fasting, your stools might also be yellow. This is because your fecal matter has been carried too rapidly down the digestive tube for the microbes to perform their miracles. No worries. Cure the diarrhea and you should eliminate the yellow color. (However, if your stools are normally bright yellow, you might consult with your physician.)

Sleep

During fasting, and especially the second day of a two day fast, I can have some difficulty with my sleep. I both have some difficulty getting to sleep and some difficulty staying asleep and/or getting back to sleep. The problem is not terrible, but is noticeable. Apparently the increase of nor-adrenalin and cortisol produced during fasting can disturb sleep. So far, my sleep problem has been handled successfully with meditation. I simply focus on a lovely, peaceful image in my mind and pull my mind back to this when it wanders. In a short while I usually have fallen asleep.

Like a Swim Bladder

The Poet's Weight Loss Plan
utilizes intermittent fasting
as a fish would
its swim bladder.

Six days a week you eat normally.
The vast majority of people
are successful at this,
as are fish at swimming horizontal.

On the seventh day you adjust:
fasting to become one pound lighter,
normal eating to remain the same.

Rather like a fish seeking to rise in fish society
by taking on a big gulp of air -
you look around, take stock of yourself
and disdain/or not from eating.

TYING THE TWO TOGETHER FOR A WINNING STRATEGY

Achieving a sustained preferred weight is a task of employing a comfortable level of self-discipline. We are creatures who eat. And we like to eat, some of us more than others. It often takes discipline to eat just what we need. And it takes even more discipline to eat less than we need. It isn't just a question of body awareness. Like I would tell my son, "What does being full have to do with it? I know I'm full. I know I'm not hungry. But this stuff is delicious." We all possess an élan vital which at times just wants to 'go for it'. You don't want to lose this 'élan vital. A good appetite is a sign of health. But it's a balance to keep our appetite under control. Our élan vital is a good concept to touch on. Because whether or not to eat that glazed donut is more of a grey area to the weight conscious than might at first be supposed.

Discipline is a tricky thing to maintain. Too strict of a discipline can foment a lapse; your 'élan vital will rebel. But too loose a discipline can lead a person to lose their way altogether. Saint Paul cautioned his brethren not to tempt sin, which can be a more powerful and clever force than they. Likewise don't tempt your 'élan vital.

There are oodles of diet plans out there, and dozens of tips upon what to eat, types of foods to avoid, when to eat, how to eat. There is a plethora of material about body type, endocrine function, genetic endowment, sex and many other contributing factors to weight gain or loss. But as my internal medicine doctor carefully explained to me: scientific experiments have shown that people who are overweight, are overweight because they eat more calories than they require. Fat is not made out of air. It is made out of food. If you eat more calories in a day, than the number of calories your body burns in a day, you will gain weight.

Over the past year I have been able to lose one pound per week regularly by eating a Diabetes Type 2 diet and fasting every Wednesday. (When Wednesday proved impossible, I moved it to Thursday. And then, when I needed to progress faster, I began fasting both days.) That's my diet. So why am I writing a book? Well, you can't market two sentences. Also 'the devil is in the details'.

Luckily, Exercise Does Not Play a Major Role in Weight Loss

Luckily, exercise does not play a major role in weight loss,
because I like to sit
and read
and think
and pet my dog
and look around.

I do not want to be the fellow running past bare-chested
with his trim, blonde, pony-tail-pulled-through-the-back-cap-band
vixen prancing at his side
like a thoroughbred show horse
in pink.
I don't mind at all being the fellow watching
and not having to keep up.
And I don't like running around with my shirt off.
If I'm going with my shirt off,
it'll be by the pool
sitting with a beer
watching the women with a little more flesh
jiggling and moving a bit more
languorously.

I do not want to be the fellow
swinging from a rock wall,
hanging from gliders,
laying a new patio,
removing that widow maker from atop of that 60 foot tree,
or fighting crime, fires, ISIS,
or even going to the moon.
Because
I like to sit
and read
and think
and pet my dog
and look around.

And a major detail is this. *The Poet's Weight Loss Plan* is a matter of one hand helping the other. When we become hungry for progress, we fast, and when we become famished for food, we eat. It can't be more natural nor made simpler.

How Slender Are We Going to Be?

We old walruses
whistling into the wind
through our yellowing tusks,
ask this of our diet program.

There is no need to appear formidable,
but lithe, agile, and fleet
are pleasing adjectives.

I want my Panama shirt to hang freely
and for my food to fall to the ground.
Every seat belt should snap loosely.
I don't want Poochie stomach.

I want to be able to bend in the middle,
something like an articulated bus.
(17 degrees would be fine.)

No visible cellulite! No crepe skin.
No droops nor sags,
nor flaps nor folds.

EXERCISE

No weight loss plan would be complete without mentioning the importance of regular exercise, but not because exercise will particularly help you to lose weight. A person who exercises moderately everyday for 30 minutes will only burn about 300 calories/day. This is about two teaspoons of mayonnaise and three artichoke hearts per day, or one six pack of Oreo cookies. This isn't nothing. But this amount of calorie burn is not going to lose you much fat anytime soon. The benefits of exercise are better health overall.

Regular exercise will tone and shape your body. It will produce muscle from the food you eat as the fat is lost. Inherent in *The Poet's Weight Loss Plan* is a mild yo-yoing. During the fasting period your body will eat both fat and muscle. Regular exercise will cause your body to restore this muscle during your days of regular eating.

Regular exercise also creates a positive routine, decreases appetite, elevates your mood and occupies the mealtime. Regular exercise and fitness bolster us against shocks, and naturally increases our self-discipline. Moreover, as you lose weight it's important to feel and enjoy the changes in your body. Exercise will help you to move easier, bend easier, stoop easier, and feel lighter on your feet. Losing fat can be more than looking better.

A Natural Stomach Reduction

I was eating a good-sized plate of food
at my nephew's birthday,
when I realized my stomach hurt,
actually *ached* from the stuffing.

Like a boa constrictor
who's been dormant in the wall
and must limber up the old tube
on small mice,
fasting for two days
shrinks a stomach naturally.

You dream a double cheeseburger,
but it's best to begin with the biscuit.
Move up to a few peas, some sliced ham
and a glass of water.
Rest, before slithering out to gobble that poodle
and the small baby.

MAKING PROGRESS

In the 'Muddle', Right There in the Abdomen

The middle is the hardest part of anything large. You're neither excited with the newly hatched plan and eager to begin, nor buoyed by the clear vision of completion. Instead, you're somewhere in the muddle, seemingly having lost the clearly focused enthusiasm of a journey's beginning and any sight of the hoped for end. Problems and distractions have arisen. Perhaps you've encountered your first 'set point' at around 20 pounds down. And whether or not the mission is even possible might now seem a matter of conjecture, probabilities and 'up for grabs'. The middle of anything large is a region of growing doubts of all sorts.

But the middle is also that area where the solution begins to manifest. A practical resolve starts to assemble itself out of the fog. What the 'muddle' in the middle actually represents is the *negotiation period*. A lot of life tends from the middle, and a lot of the body rotates around it. *The Poet's Weight Loss Plan* certainly does. The middle is where the "rubber meets the road" and there is no getting around it - there is only the going through it. It is from this 'muddle' that your new, actual lifestyle will emerge.

Seemingly a large portion of people don't make it much past the beginning of a diet. Many people adopt an 'all or nothing' attitude towards their dieting. They set themselves an extraordinarily hard goal and/or give up at the first sign of failure. For example, finding that they've habitually reached for and eaten a cookie, they then toss up their hands and eat the whole box.

Inadequate sleep can make us feel hungrier. (Plus we're awake longer to act upon this.)

Irregular meal schedules play havoc with plans.

Other studies suggest people fail at diets because their diets:

1) deprive
2) are temporary
3) don't fit with normal life
4) are expensive
5) they can lower our metabolism
6) must be combined with exercise.

No surprises here. But studies also suggest that people who will succeed: start and are persistent, see failure as something to expect, and

Losing Weight is *Hard*

Examining the numbers,
we have found
that sustained weight loss is half as hard as
becoming a Navy Seal.
Or conversely,
half of those who achieve sustained weight loss
are statistically
tough as Navy Seals.

But that was then,
and this is now.
With *The Poet's Weight Loss Plan*
we have devised a self-customizing boot camp
which adjusts like an elastic band
to the weight loss rate you can sustain.

Imagine having to swim
500 yards breaststroke in under 9 minutes
as a Navy Seal is required to do -
but having as long a time as you need to do it!
This is basically what *The Poet's Weight Loss Plan's*
'customized difficulty feature' ® achieves.
We are like dripping water on a flabby rock.
You can achieve a Navy Seal's distinction with this:
The Poet's Weight Loss Plan

 'Fat is not an option.'

Why are you waiting?

"put on their hard hats" - that is, they follow their plan no matter how they might feel at the time. This is what self-discipline is: the ability to do what needs doing irrespective of how we feel.

Losing a large amount of weight is no different from any other large project. It takes a long period of time. The advance is incremental as the diversions grow. The discipline while growing established can also grow worn, and stretched out of strict conformity. It is hard to stay focused for such a long period of time. There needs to be something in the action itself which provides the focus; which is always in motion, creating direction like a gyroscope. In a marriage, this is the love engendered through the experiences that accrue through time. It supplies momentum. For a successful diet, the practitioner must create the same sort of gyroscopic mechanism from the elements of their habit. What is there about a dietary discipline which causes it to sustain itself?

Midway through my plan I hit a slippery patch. Somewhere between 20 - 30 pounds lost (it was hard to know) my scale weights were either wrong, or I wasn't losing, or I was eating more than I'd thought, or the weight of my clothes was effecting the outcome. I didn't seem to be losing weight as I should, or maybe I was but it wasn't showing? I didn't know. But I didn't quit the diet. And the reason I didn't quit the diet was that I had found a reasonable eating arrangement which worked for me. I didn't want to change how I ate. It was comfortable, and doable. *There was really nothing to quit!* I hadn't gained weight. So I just continued on. This, to me, marks a successful diet. At this point, all I needed to do was to take a breath, let a little time pass and to tease out what exactly was going on and then make the needed adjustments - if I wanted to.

The Poet's Weight Loss Plan's insight is to combine a situation in which people are quite successful, that is, normal eating, with the situation in which people are most motivated, that is, losing weight as fast as possible. We obtain our sustained weight loss goal by enjoying our success in both of these situations. We simply trim one's normal eating of fast-acting carbohydrates and excessive portions. And the person gets to lose their weight as fast as is possible by fasting - but only for the duration of a day (or two), which is statistically a length of caloric restriction nearly everyone can finish. People enjoy being successful. They enjoy meeting their goals. They enjoy pride. And they want to enjoy this as much as possible. The Poet's Weight Loss Plan offers you the enjoyment of daily success. It is in the workings and negotiations of the middle ground where the poise of your daily rituals will be found. And you can do this successfully.

...with Pickle Spear

I was so infatuated by the phrase *'with pickle spear'*
attached to the end
of a humdrum sandwich selection,
like the garnish it is,
on the clear coated lunchroom menu.
that I just *had* to say it!

"I didn't get my *pickle spear*.
Each sandwich is supposed to come with "fries,
or a bag of chips, and... *'with pickle spear'*."
I glanced about with delight,
mouthing the phrase,
as if to remark to all,
through a conductor's wave of my arms,
that
'I'm not really complaining.
I don't really care! '
'Whatever!'

For what was later brought out
by the waitress,
on a single white plate:
a single spear of pickle,
of singular importance,
looking like *nouvelle cuisine*.

No one knew quite what to make of
such enthusiasm for a *pickle spear*...
which proposed to claim a phalanx of waiters.
My wife was perhaps a little embarrassed.

And I wonder,
if people could find this,
that is me,
a little confusing?

The Set Point Theory

A mystery can be like muddy water. If you wait a while, the situation will clear. In my situation it seems what I had encountered was my body's first metabolic *set point*. Though not proven, set point theory is a widely held belief in the weight loss community. The set point theory maintains that each of us has a weight set point above or below which the body will adjust metabolically, hormonally and behaviorally to regain what your body believes to be your necessary weight. This is your body's set point. A personal set point is as individual as facial appearance. Some of us have low set points and stay slender. Some of us have high set points and tend to be overweight and remain so. *But your set point can change with time.* (I wasn't born weighing 315 pounds!)

Evolutionary survival is hypothesized to have made us so that set point rise occurs much more easily than set point decrease. Factors such as over eating, age, lack of activity, high caloric diets and artificial sweeteners which change the gut flora, can all raise an individual's set point. Factors such as sustained physical exercise and testosterone, spicy foods, exercise change-ups, are believed to be able to lower a person's set point. But the most natural way a person's set point can lower is over time through slow, steady weight loss.

A therapist, who has made it their practice to work with people to lose between 100 - 200 pounds naturally, states that this weight loss usually takes the client between 3 - 5 years. And during this time the patient will hit weight loss plateaus at various points for individual patients. When a patient hits a weight loss plateau, this is evidence that the patient has encountered set point resistance. *The fix is to maintain the slow steady dieting until the body "settles in" to a new (lower) set point.* This can take from 6-8 weeks to occur. After this time, regular weight loss will again occur while dieting.

Dieting without weight loss can be a daunting thing. But knowing that this phenomenon is to be expected, that no one escapes it, and that simply continuing the diet will resolve the problem all help to get a person through it. A great advantage is when the dieter has achieved a peace with their diet such that they will have no trouble sustaining it forever. For this person, the weight loss plateau offers little difficulty. When there's no end, a little bit of delay makes little difference.

For this reason, it is fortunate if your set point plateau does not occur until you have been dieting for 4-5 months and have reached a reasonable

This Diet

is like a jade plant,
which requires only occasional care.
You needn't examine nor weigh it, everyday.
It's best kept out of the light,
out of the way,
perhaps on a book shelf
next to the home remedies and practical medicine.

It could be happy as a member of the kitchen,
perhaps kept on a sideboard.
It grows slowly, is quietly sustaining,
and takes its greatest sustenance from the air,
from the mood, and the general ambience actually.

Unostentatious as a can of soup,
and seemingly as odd
in these days of overconsumption and rapid eating
 - do not overfeed nor overwater.
It's leaves and stems have the survival skills, and
the rich, waxy, big, green plumpness
of a quiet resolve.

peace with expectations. One way to insure that you are ready to meet the challenge of your set point plateau is to move slowly and gradually by fasting only one day / week.

Priorities

All strategies have priorities. Evidence demonstrates that when the #1 priority is weight loss, the chances of failure are near 100%. ***Your #1 priority should be continuing the diet plan.*** Anyone who continues with this diet plan will succeed.

The #2 priority is to maintain a level of self-discipline necessary to succeed at #1. We do this by resting 6 days a week.

The #3 priority is weight loss based on sound nutrition. If the two first priorities are met, this third will follow. It needn't be coaxed.

When you eat nutritiously and take in less calories/day than you burn, weight loss *will* occur.

Use an Accurate Home Scale

Five months into my diet I had lost 20 pounds. Three more weeks into my diet I had lost only 21 pounds, even though I had begun fasting two days/week in order to speed the process. This was quite distressing. I had been feeling very comfortable with my ability to control my eating, because the diet had the latitude in portion size, quality, simplicity and special occasion eating, to make me feel I could continue with it for the rest of my life. Now it seemed, by my calculations, that I had been eating 1500 calories/day too much! This was terrible! Cutting out 1500 calories/day would destroy the comfort and confidence I had with my current eating. I could do it. But I couldn't imagine sustaining it. And if I could not sustain the eating side of my diet, the whole plan would not work.

We repeat: Fasting is easy; eating is hard.

Fortunately or unfortunately, as it turned out, I had used a scale in my father-in-law's cardiologist's office to weigh myself. So I decided to place new batteries in my scale at home and measure my weight again on the home scale, just in the off chance that the fancy scale at the cardiologist's was wrong. Relief! I had actually lost around 4.5 lbs., which, though it was

An Overweight Sherlock Holmes Takes on Set Point Theory

It's alimentary my dear Watson;
this one thing leading to the next.
The set point hates change.
It wants me today,
just as I was yesterday.
If my internal metabolism could wear epaulettes,
a shiny cap and wave a riding crop,
it would.

And really, such hidebound behavior is in need
of a quick attitude adjustment to my mind.
I control my mouth, hands and lips.
I'm not eating more calories than I burn each day,
until one or the other of us snaps!
And then, that'll be the end of it,

Granted, I'm messing with my Set Point.
But mind you, it's just a theory.
So if its feelings are hurt,
where's the harm?

Let's see how my petty little inner mind martinet likes this
yesterday,
tomorrow,
and then the day after?
I don't think my Set Point has the grit to stick it out, actually.
It likes consistency too much.

not the 6 lbs. I had programmed to lose, was still respectable. I had binged a bit, and this was not unexpected.

The takeaway here is that even modern, expensive looking digital scales in doctor's offices can vary several pounds in their readings from other scales. So weigh yourself with the same home scale each time, wearing the same amount of clothing (or not), and at the same day of the week and time of day.

Weight Loss Depression

About midway through my diet my limbs had slimmed, my neck and face were slimmer, and I had begun to lose the tummy bump. But I found myself becoming glum. It just seemed I had gotten depressed about the whole project without a reason why - other than midway through anything is a tough section of roadway. I figured it was something just to be expected and to stay the course, to just soldier on and the feeling would pass.

The feeling did pass. But the feeling passed as a realization dawned. I realized one day as I mulled the situation over, that when I had imagined myself back at the weight I was at the age of 30, that I was viewing myself as I was then. But when I looked into the mirror - instead, I looked *old* (presently 70). And it struck me that no matter how much weight lost, I would still look *old*. I would never be the youth of my imagination.

Eventually my depression passed into a pretty river rock. As a poet friend used to say of each job or situation he was either fired from or left: "Well, there's a pretty good poem in that."

As I took stock in the fog of my rather slight depression, I realized that my weight gain over the years had also been my ace in the hole. Without telling myself as much, I had let myself emotionally assume that the changes of age could be reversed when I had finally decided to get serious, to put the hammer down and lose weight. This didn't happen. The best that happened was that I lost weight.

The worse that happens is that slender people look even older than fat ones! In terms of age I had lost even more ground.

You might have noticed that I depend upon strategy a lot to negotiate life, and that a large portion of my strategizing involves perspective. This is

Going Without Food

the first day is like a partial eclipse.
The daylight is dimmer but
you can still see the food shining brightly
where it covers the refrigerator glass,
the bread box, the cabinet shelves, and here and there
sprinkled across the table and counters in dappled
arrangement.

The second day comes with greater tedium,
watching time's procession of missed meals,
like empty big rigs passing,
deadheading to their next engagement.
The rigs move lighter, climb the hills better,
but there is no reward
and the drivers shuffle country songs,
antsy to get on with it.

And then, somehow
 - and you're not quite certain how it would work -
but fasting *feels* as if it should involve some eating.
Just as marriage *feels* at times as if it should involve
some cheating.
Let your brain chew on that.
But don't trust anything it comes up with.

true. And what I finally decided upon was to change my goal. I decided that the look of a scrappy, lean, seventy year old with close cropped hair could still work. I would replace my youth with poise. Poise can accumulate with age. And being slender has a look of poise. And when I wear my gray hair short, shave, (especially the ear and nose hairs), keep myself clean and dress with fashion, then add the seasoned voice of age and so far the feedback has been good.

People notice the weight loss and say I look "great". Who am I to argue?

Renewing Our Vows

Each weekly fast renews our vows. Each week our level of discipline is reset. Fasting eradicates laxity. It's an entirely binary decision with no grey area. You are back on the wagon, where no excuses are accepted and no slack cut.

Few persons can maintain the strictures of a diet over a great length of time. (Like permanently.) But many people can diet for a week. This is what we are doing. We are dieting for one week - over and over again.

Your Personal Discipline is a Fragile Thing

I swim for exercise six days a week, one half mile, twenty two laps of the pool. Two years into this regimen it's gotten easy. But I'm hesitant to increase either the length or the intensity of the regimen. It's easy on most days, but it's just doable on the bad days. And it's the bad days that my personal discipline is calibrated for, because my number one priority is not to quit doing my regular exercise. And so far, for two years, I haven't quit.

Your personal dietary discipline can be a fragile thing also. Guard it. Letting other needs muscle it out can kill it. Bragging about it can kill it. Being greedy and pushing for more can stack too much upon its spindly legs. Your personal discipline's most important measure is its persistence. There is a good reason alcoholics don't judge themselves upon how *much* alcohol they've refused and instead judge themselves upon how long it's been since their last drink.

For many reasons, some conscious and some unconscious, you have a level of discipline you have managed to commit to. Be very careful with it,

Devouring Cold Watermelon in This Anonymous River Town

Big, oblong, and mottled green,
flat and faded yellow on the bottom
where they've sat in the field, heavy with promise -
they wobble in the back on the drive home
and respond with a ripe 'crack' as they're sliced open.

You can eat a car trunk full of all that water and fiber;
fill up for a few calories and practice a wild gluttony.
The land never felt so generous as you gaze across those
green orbs
in a hazy summer field wavering in the sun.
And as the juice dribbles from your lips onto the thirsty soil,
you know it's true that only a fool
would pass by this area's fine, vine ripened produce.

In a river bottom town,
half a watermelon should sit in the fridge
nearby a dozen cold beers, or you simply
do not have the supplies to be neighborly.

as it can be ruined. Change it a bit and it's not the discipline you managed before; you're in a new marriage without the long history of commitment. And your new discipline is vulnerable to change, followed by more change, and then another change. Without intending so, you may have altered your personal discipline into more than you can now manage. It's a tricky thing. You may not realize your loss until you have failed. Guard your personal discipline, as if it were your wife. They can be more fragile than you might think.

Arrogance

There's always a fly in the ointment, and they really collect around weight loss.

The particular fly of *arrogance* would seem to make its appearance at around 25-30 pounds of weight loss. At 10 pounds people are usually feeling pretty good about themselves and pleased with their progress and others are pleased with them. Part of the reason for this is that the 'other' people have been down this road and suspect that a bit of time will make their 'slim' neighbor 'fat' again. This is usually the case.

At 25-30 pounds weight loss the dieter may have seen such obvious changes in their physique as to feel confident and prideful. Arrogance arrives shortly thereafter. (Don't look at me. I didn't create Original Sin.)

It's a near certainty that at some point you will begin to associate all sorts of fine and rare character traits to yourself as you see your thinning self to be more and more elect. This is illusory! All you have done is to lose some weight. You have not saved lives, defended your country, or slaved at a desk job or in the home for forty years to raise children and then put them through college. All you have done is to shrink! You've gotten *smaller*. Don't start staring down your spectacles at plump people.   Celebrate, but keep it in proportion. Always remember, when the *ugly green urge* to judge others slithers out to speak, "There but for the Grace of God waddles me."

The Ugly Green Urge Replies

(Here at the Poet's Corner we respect freedom of speech. So without further comment I include this reply from the smug.)

Bad Dream #2

Fat people fly upwards
generating fat shadows
bending across pizzas and hot dog stands
and darkening Big Gulps
as they eclipse the sun.

The children sweat and wheeze as they waddle forth
to line up for ice cream.
Great dirigibles of hamburgers and candy bars
fill the air, also,
casting huge darknesses over the fair.

"Isn't it pretty to think so?" Hemingway wrote, as a last line to *The Sun Also Rises*. It will also serve as a first line to this retort:

The truth of the matter is that one of the prime determinants of whether a person will succeed at the dieting or not, is whether the discipline will achieve for the dieter a sought ethos, which Google defines as, "the characteristic spirit of a culture, era, or community as manifested in its beliefs and aspirations." In other words, most of us strongly aspire to achieve membership in our desired social grouping, and we are willing to do a lot to accomplish this. Personally, I did not want to look like a fraud when my diet book came out, and honestly this provided much motivation to persevere. Likewise, it is undeniable that many, if not most of the friends I've known, who manage to stay quite trim throughout their latter years, fairly obviously exhibit quite a bit of resolve to do so. ("What's a guy got to do to get something to eat around here?" being one of my major complaints when visiting with them.) Being slim in our society is a hallmark of the upper classes. And it's such an obvious hallmark (your physique is like a walking billboard of your cultural status) that parading it about can be quite intoxicating for the status conscious. (Which to some extent, includes us all.) So, in short, being 'smug' about your trim looks will go a long way in helping you to maintain them.

So, it only makes sense to utilize the energies released by the 'green urge of arrogance'. Go ahead: be prideful. Be smug. But remember, just like with their wealth, the upper classes do not flaunt. *If you want class; have some class.* Your smugness should be understated, as to appear something you're hardly aware of, like the pleasant fragrance of an expensive perfume. "Yes. Of course," you might agree. "I'm blessed with good genes."

But, if your smugness does keep the fatties away - so much the better. That's more celery for yourself.

Vacation and Holiday Setbacks

It's easy to take a vacation and return home to realize you've gained 10-20 pounds. You've tried to continue your reasonable eating habits and yet, there it is - or seems to be. Take a deep breath. Things may not be as dire as they seem. This has happened to me, also.

Recently I took a ten day vacation and when I weighed myself upon my return, I had gained ten pounds! Sure, I had let myself enjoy some time off.

Stereotyping

At times during my *Poet's Weight Loss Plan* ©
 I have personified my fat,
as if I were just going through
a messy divorce.
Which, of course, was a way of falsifying
her
unknowable nature.

But I was reasonable sure that there was just no way I had eaten a pounds worth of extra fat per day!

As it worked out, the weight came off nearly as fast. When we eat either more or less on a fairly regular basis, for a brief period of time, great shifts of fluid volume take place. We discussed earlier how the beginning dieter is falsely cheered by the ease with which they can lose their first 10-15 pounds. And that this is due mostly to the loss of fluids, waste and digestive juices.

When back from your vacation, get back on your regular dietary program, and your weight should re-adjust itself nearly as quickly. There may be only two or three pounds of actual fat which you've acquired.

My Mouth Cries

*"...fasting,
my spirit descends into Hades"*
- Paul Baryne

Fasting has the loneliness of the widower.
Once you get good at fasting,
it's not the hunger so much
as missing food.

Like a widower breathing in his wife's pillow -
you miss that warm, fragrant
arrangement on the plate,
the heaping forkful of it.

The smells are almost a meal.
I relish the time spent
seating myself,
bringing on the dish,
warming my nose in the vapors,
like watching my wife
prepare for bed.

The crunch and the swallow,
the gulp and belch,
my mouth tears up
and the gut begins to howl
from missing my dinner friend.
A fast leaves so much of me bereft.

THINGS I'VE NOTICED

Wild Horses

Everything likes to eat. Take wild horses, for example, roaming the vacant West, racing up canyons or across rolling grasslands exuberant in their freedom. But how do we find them most of the time? Most of the time, we find them eating grass and browsing before a grand view like the wealthy on their patios. If you like to eat and have a good appetite, you're healthy. Eating is natural.

I've come to think that overeating is natural also. My experience with this diet would indicate that I am most comfortable in my eating when I am eating somewhat more than a day's allotment in calories. This seems to allow me a latitude in my choices, portions and indulgences which suits me like loose clothing (which is how I prefer to dress). I can stick with this diet quite comfortably. But, it means also that I must fast one day per week, to maintain my weight. This may well have been the eating situation in our early evolution - more than adequate game and nutrition for several days, and then nothing for a day. Or, maybe I just like to think so.

Marriage

Everything you do in a marriage affects your spouse. Even losing weight affects the equilibrium. But you can be the leader. Without criticizing, you may provide your mate with some of your strength to lean on. They will appreciate it.

Swimming

When you're overweight, swimming is a good way to exercise without undue wear and tear on the joints. Right away, your total weight becomes that minus the weight of a like volume of water, so your total weight is that of a dehydrated you, a totally desiccated you. In fact, it would be fun to weigh oneself in the water to see what that weight would be.

As you step up those pool stairs, all that weight is accrued back, like a thoroughbred being handicapped. It would also be interesting to have a scale on each step to measure better the feel of the addition of pounds.

Refrigerator Poem / "I'm Saving This for My Diet"

This poem is all about me.
It's not about you,
or you,
or you...

I'm going to buy what I like,
and place it where I like,
for my own enjoyment,
as long as I like.

You have neither been consulted, nor considered.
I don't care about your mother,
or if love has treated you roughly.
Perhaps your dad wasn't all that he should have been.
I'm not gonna entertain it here.

And don't touch anything!
Leave it just. as. is.

Overweight, we are like race horses operating far below our best, eating the dust of our not-so-betters without the weight sewn in their saddlebags.

Wouldn't it be nice to know at which step you will feel the weight of your diet goal, and then, to look forward to that - or, better yet, to set your diet goal at that step where you feel your best?

I'm Enjoying Weighing Less

It is important to enjoy and let yourself hope for a whole assortment of associated victories. I'm hoping to get off my Diabetes Type 2 medication, and to have my glucose test normal. I'm hoping to dispense with my hypertension and cholesterol medication. It would be fine to eliminate most of the medication I take. It would be especially nice if losing the weight actually cured these other conditions. These are associated goals and victories to keep in mind.

I would feel proud to have managed a feat many people cannot.

I also am enjoying weighing less. My face is slimmer. My stomach does not hang over my belt. My pants do not slip down. I bend easier. I have a small and quiet sense of pride walking my dog about the neighborhood. Pride in that I have found a way to accomplish weight loss, which I have wanted to accomplish, and it is happening. And I am feeling in charge of how I want to appear.

What gives me the greatest confidence is that through some lapse and inconsistencies in my normal eating habits, I have recorded the same weight loss week by week. (Excepting for those set point plateaus. But they are temporary.) *Probably the most gratifying feeling is of the control I feel that I can decide the weight I want to be and then sustain it. No more hopelessness.*

Traditional Discipline

The Poet's Weight Loss Plan
is a disciplined player of the long game
who embed themselves within
the day to day proprieties
so that when opportunity comes along
they're church ready.

Nothing controls the mood like tradition.
Gargantuan proportions,
like silicon enhanced breasts,
represent the collapse of all dignity.

It is important to observe this:
that poise and eating go hand in hand.
Proper table manners bespeak proper upbringing
which bespeak proper portions.
And established custom
requires little discipline.

AND FINALLY, CONCERNS

Intermittent fasting, as it is practiced here, is safe and is one of the world's best weight loss tools. Intermittent fasting has been shown to not decrease your metabolism nor induce more than a mild compensatory eating backlash. *During fasting of up to 48 hours the body's metabolism has been shown to actually increase. Intermittent fasting also has been shown to cause a much smaller amount of muscle loss that conventional dietary calorie restriction.*

Fasting for a day or two (Also known as the 5:2 diet or "The Fast Diet".) is rarely a problem for a healthy individual. However, it could be dangerous if you are someone with kidney or liver problems, immunological problems or are not regularly eating a healthy diet. Also, whereas fasting is generally not a problem for persons on most medications, each medication varies and the absorption, activity, and other effects of medication can vary with a fast. It is prudent to check with your doctor and to read your medication inserts.

Fasting might also affect your blood pressure, but it's hard to state firmly which way. Though I am fasting in order to lose weight and lower my blood pressure, during the fast it has sometimes increased by 20mm/systolic and 10mm diastolic while on my hypertensive medication and by even more when off. My research indicates that blood pressure is generally supposed to go down during fasting. But people also report that while fasting their blood pressure rose. My blood pressure over the past year while fasting has gone both directions. At any rate the blood pressure rise has not been so great as to place me anywhere near danger. My advice is that if you have concerns about your blood pressure while using this diet, keep a blood pressure monitor at your desk. Monitor it closely. If something concerns you, consult your doctor. If you are on blood pressure medication, you might also consult your doctor before fasting, as the electrolyte depletion produced by fasting can be additional to that caused by prescribed diuretics. This can increase your chance of fainting.

Certain people shouldn't fast. These include:*
  - Pregnant women
  - People with wasting diseases or malnutrition

Lunches I've Dreamed of

Nothing marks us like a dream.
With me, a ham on cheese always predominates,
with lettuce, mayonnaise, a sun-ripened tomato slice
on raisin bread and cut in half diagonally
on a small plate with chips,
the crunchy artisanal kind.

I'm not a major player.
I fashion a dream, and then I eat it.
What could be simpler, less cumbersome?
Leaving only a few crumbs, but no burnt villages
with their fleeing populations,
nor effort-filled years of ego gratifications
abandoned or receding into oblivion.

A ham sandwich, like a poem, is a noon's work;
clean, tasty - maybe with a little mustard - and easily
digested.
Quick and fleeting, evanescent,
ham with a tangy garnish
are love words
melding back into existence -
small, humble, satisfying. Chew it,
and you're done.

- Someone with a history of cardiac arrhythmias
  People with hepatic or renal insufficiency.

*(Fuhrman http://www.webmd.com/diet/features/is_fasting_healthy#1)

The diabetic medication, Metaformin's, effects are not unduly influenced by fasting. But if you take other forms of diabetic medication, you should discuss its use during fasting and whether fasting is safe for you with your doctor. Many people simply adjust the dosage.

When breaking your fast, especially after a two day fast, do not indulge. Give your digestive tract a little time to adjust. Maybe cut that wonderful breakfast you envisioned in half. Eat one half at breakfast, and the other a couple hours later as your snack.

Of special caution: Use prudence in the hot tub or sauna on fasting days and the day after. I found, especially during the second day's fast, that soaking in the hot tub after my swim could lead to a fairly severe faintness upon leaving the pool. It could be several minutes before I felt steady enough to head to the shower. I would especially caution anyone who is diabetic, elderly or suffering from any sort of heart problem.

On a follow up note, however, I found that after taking replacement electrolyte capsules (one at the time of each missed meal with a big glass of water), fainting was not a problem. (See previous section on *Diarrhea and Hypotension*.)

Diabetic Ketoacidosis

The body normally produces ketones in response to fasting.

Diabetic Ketoacidosis is a relatively rare occurrence in fasting persons with Type 2 Diabetes. However, it is a danger for people with Type 1 Diabetes. Fasting during an infection or illness or while taking steroids can increase the risks as the body becomes more insulin resistant during these times. Or it might occur in people yet undiagnosed with Type 1 Diabetes.

Diabetic ketoacidosis occurs when there is not enough insulin produced by the body. The fat cells keep releasing fat into the bloodstream which the liver then converts into ketones and ketoacids. This causes a lowering of the blood pH (ketoacidosis).

Spicy Chicken Wings

If you overeat these
and you are like me,
there's a good chance you've eaten
far, far, far too many.

The tub of chicken wings is gone.
There is no need to look.
You can feel your nails
scratching the bare cardboard.

This horse has left the barn,
or flown the coop, as it were.
And you will not desire another gallon
of greasy chicken wings
for several years.

This problem is somewhat
self-limiting.

Symptoms of DKA include:

- Nausea, vomiting
- Stomach pain
- Fruity breath – the smell of ketoacids
- Frequent urination
- Excessive thirst
- Weakness, fatigue
- Speech problems, confusion or unconsciousness
- Heavy, deep breathing

https://dtc.ucsf.edu/living-with-diabetes/complications/diabetic-ketoacidosis/

There's a double-edged sword here. When you metabolize fat you create ketones and ketoacids. So if you intend to lose fat, you will create a certain level of ketosis. What is important to remember is that the body is an extremely complex high wire act of competing processes through which it practices the 'middle way'. Be aware of symptoms of the extreme, and when they appear do what your body would do - take appropriate measures.

If you should develop ketoacidosis, you should discontinue your fast and see a doctor. You might be pushing your fasting too hard, or you might have an undiagnosed condition or a condition that poses more restrictions than you had realized.

Like Anything Else

Dieting is like anything else.
You will lose weight faster,
once you get good at it.

You don't get right on a bike
and ride twenty-five miles.
In your first five months
you may lose twenty pounds.

You may have lost only twenty pounds,
but you have gotten fairly good at dieting.
Over the next five, let's lose forty.

At some point in the future
we might have to worry about
you disappearing altogether.

AND A FEW MORE THINGS

"How tough are you?" (cop)
"I'm tough enough." (private detective)

What if you are not a person with much self-discipline, or feel that you are not?

There are two answers to this. The first is that self-discipline is like a muscle, and every time you exercise self-discipline, you strengthen this muscle. The second is that the key to possession of the required self-discipline is *strategy*. You must adopt a strategy which comes closest to requiring the most comfortable amount of self-discipline you can muster. *In other words, rather than structuring this diet around rate of weight loss, we structure it to match your self-discipline.* The important thing is to be 'tough enough'.

How about a diet which requires no self-discipline?

There is no such thing. To lose weight requires the body to take in less calories than it needs. Your body will fight this. To maintain the weight which you achieve will require you to forego eating excessive calories. We not only eat to fulfill our need for food, but we often like to eat more than we need. You will want two cookies instead of one. A certain amount of self-discipline is necessary for success. So, we'd best go about building a successful strategy.

Now I am not a person who is very good at the brilliant win, and that is what credentials are often about. But I am pretty good at playing the long game. In the long game, played at the highest level, there is no winning... as there is no end. What the long game entails are strategies which keep you playing. Staying alive, achieving an MD degree, telemarketing, writing, poetry, being married with children - all of which I've done - all require long game strategies. Sustained weight loss is this sort of game. If you don't see yourself as a 'winner', you might think that you won't have much success at sustained weight loss. The opposite could very well be the case. People who demand big wins often quit, quickly.

Weight Poem

It would be stupid to write a book
and not learn something.
And then, after you've learned something,
not to alter course a bit,

so that the plan grows
like a plant.
The top does not look like the roots
nor exactly any portion of the plan in between.

It's not uncommon for a plant
to end in a flower.
There's the payload.
So too, it's a good idea,
if you do decide it's a good book,
to read the book to its end.

The conclusion this book reaches
may delight and surprise you.
Use it to decorate your head.

EPILOGUE

The Poet's (Forty Pound) Weight Loss Plan

"Before you heal someone, ask him if he's willing to give up the things which make him sick."

- Hippocrates

Over eighteen months, I lost 45 pounds. I had intended to lose fifty pounds before finishing this book and calling it "The Poet's Weight Loss Plan". There is good reason for trying out your ideas first. Experience holds many more surprises than we imagine. The first surprise for me was that whereas my weight at 315 pounds might be generally maintained with simple prudent eating - my weight at 270 pounds would not.

How do I know this? I tried it.

My weight loss hit a wall at 45 pounds lost. I found I was fasting two days/week just to remain at weight. I tried upping it to fasting three days/week. But my family rebelled. I was becoming too irritable to be around, like that fellow in the Snickers commercial. So I decided I would not completely fast, but would eat just enough food in small amounts so as to not feel hunger and try to continue losing weight that way. Two things happened: I soon began eating larger snacks. And I did not lose any more weight. So I decided, since it was fall and the holidays were coming, I would simply eat comfortably - continuing with my diabetes Type 2 regimen - and weigh myself again, after several months, to see whether or not my weight loss was sustained.

This brings me to my current situation, which is an appropriate place for this book to end.

A good life requires poise and self-discipline. A person cannot do whatever they feel like doing and have things work out well. I cannot allow myself to eat as would most please me, and maintain my weight. The reason we find so many people explaining that they are on a diet - is because that is what it takes to maintain a weight, which is a continual awareness of one's weight and how many calories they are taking in. It needn't be overwhelming, but it is something that will have to be somewhere on your mind all of the time, rather like knowing, if only in a general way, where your kids might be.

Fortieth Pound

If you lose weight in a forest
are you lighter?
If I drank more water,
would that help?
"To be or not to be, that is the question."
The meal branched after the soup,
and I took the one less ordered,
and that has made all the difference.
Less is more.

This shouldn't come as a big surprise. We don't stay in shape without regular exercise. We don't naturally like to exert ourselves. Even Balanchine remarked that he had to continually badger his dancers to get them to move. And movement was their chosen profession!

And so it is with weight. Maintaining the weight you chose will be a regular, ongoing commitment. Just as a person must make themselves go to the gym regularly; so must a person watch their eating.

After two years, I know my way around the Diabetes Type 2 diet fairly well. I've also become fairly adept at fasting. It's no big thing to not eat for a day.

So I weigh myself weekly; adjusting my diet and eating to maintain a forty pound loss.

Why forty pounds? There are a number of reasons, just as there will be number of reasons for the weight you finally choose to be, or which chooses you.

Reason number one is that 275 pounds seems to be a weight I can maintain. There are lots of exercise plans a person can adopt. But the most important exercise plan for the person to adopt is the one which keeps that person exercising week after week, year after year. Surely, there are many that would make a person more fit or with better cross training advantages. But instead of being all you can be for a short time, it is better to be the most you can be all of the time. Forty pounds weight loss seems to represent a sustainable weight for me.

Reason number two is that at forty pounds weight loss my blood glucose index is in the normal range. This is necessary. I also no longer snore. This is quite pleasant for my wife.

Reason number three is that at forty pounds weight loss I have regained most of my ordinary flexibility. I can bend over to pick up the dog's droppings without undo difficulty. I can pick up something dropped on the floor without swearing too loudly.

Reason number four is that at forty pounds weight loss I look good (enough), and my clothes fit fairly well. I'm still an older male with a bit of flab, but I embrace it. It's a benchmark of living successfully as long as I have.

Reason number five is that I now compare people's builds, their activity level and how they eat. I do not want to spend more time exercising than 30 minutes a day, six days a week. I don't want to do marathon runs or endurance triathlons. I also want to eat more than the skeletal people I see browsing over small plates of vegetables and tofu cubes. When I recall

Un-Fortunate Cookies

Cookie #1
Your private indulgence
has grown public
and is flopping about provocatively.

Cookie #2
Fat weighs you down
in your climb
to the top.

Cookie #3
Your personal brand
is huffing and puffing.

XXXL Cookie #4
Sweaty and lugubrious
as a Chinese autocrat
stuffed with greasy pressed duck
and sticky rice...

your fat is like a potentate
of the Middle Kingdom
with his elastics and gussets
living large in the midst of things.

the people I know, or have known, who stay slender but still eat reasonably, they appear to maintain their weight by eating one healthy meal a day. And I have tired of the extremes of fasting over this period of time. Combined with small regularly spaced snacks, one right sized meal/day might well be my regimen as my journey reaches its apotheosis and my weight stabilizes where chosen.

I like to sit and reflect, and I like to eat yummy food. At 270 pounds it looks like I can continue to do this as long as I stay within my diet strategy and exercise 30 minutes/day.

So. Weight maintenance is an ongoing task, just like brushing your teeth. Depending on your current health and your facility with the tools offered in this book you will find and remain at the weight you want. That's success, and that's poise. And that's earning your smile.

And what does it cost? Nothing!

(And that's worth a smile, too.)

So...

Kicking Away the Training Wheels
(Dieting is easier, after you've eaten something.)

The Poet's Forty Pound Weight Loss Plan strategy is that of a rock climber's chimney. The dieter places their back and hands against the eating side and braces their feet against the fasting side. By using the force of one against the other we move up the chimney until we realize the weight loss we want to accomplish. There is great personal empowerment in achieving and sustaining one's preferred weight.

But a diet - any diet - is like training wheels. The Final Frontier is kicking away those training wheels, after having created a normal eating pattern which maintains your preferred weight, which you can peddle forward on without losing your balance. Accomplishing this is a gradual process of negotiation between the two sides of your rock chimney strategy until your personal summit is achieved.

For two months, I tried eating responsibly without fasting to see what would happen. Over two months I gained twenty pounds. Calculated out, this meant that as an average, I was consuming 125% of my needed calories daily. The size of my meals proves to be my biggest hurdle in maintaining my weight. This is a tough one, but...

Yes, This Fat is Me

Thank you. I enjoyed making it.
I like fat because fat feels soft, is pliable
and happens upon you like a cat.
I find myself kneading it through thoughtful moments,
like while reading a book.

It's painful to lose your fat.
We've all lost fat and know
how painful it can be.
The hurt is real.
So it's good never to take on too much.

There's a rim of fat around my belt.
That's the part that puts away a few beers
and eats some of the rum cake at Christmas.
It's the part of me which walks out to get the paper,
then sits on a rock to read it.
Loosening my shirt and letting this bit of fat out
is like turning my dog loose;
letting it sniff a bit, run around.
And not having a little blubber
would be like having a dog
and no backyard.
Or like having no dog.
Life could get very hard.

In response, I'm adding a bit of food to my fasting side, and cutting full meals from the eating side. My wife and I enjoy dinners together. But breakfast and lunch have been replaced often by snacks, here and there - enough to still any hunger pangs. No electrolyte replacement needed. We'll see if I can't get my daily intake below 100% of required and pare off those 20 pounds. If not, then back to Plan A (the beginning), until I try to kick the training wheels again.

It may take a long time before I'm maintaining my weight with balanced days. But the enjoyments of being forty pounds lighter have resolved any quibbles. I'm all in.

CARL NELSON

Silver Lining

As I settle into the hot tub Jacuzzi,
the breasts around me begin to bob.
My bulk makes all boats rise.

APPENDIX

Carbohydrate Choice Lists

15 Grams of Carbohydrate = 1 Food Choice = 1 Serving

Bread: One Food Choice

Bagel	½ (1 oz)
Bread, reduced - calorie	slices (1.5 oz)
Bread, white, whole-wheat, pumpernickel, rye	1 slice (1 oz)
Bread sticks, crisp, 4 in x .5 in	2 (2/3 oz)
English muffin	½
Hot dog or hamburger bun	½ (1 oz)
Pita, 6 in across	½
Raisin bread, unfrosted	1 slice (1 oz)
Roll, plain, small	1 (1 oz)
Tortilla, corn, 6 in across	1
Tortilla, flour, 6 in across	1
Waffle, 4.5 in square, reduced-fat	1

Cereals and Grains: One Food Choice

Bran cereals	½ cup
Cereals, unsweetened, ready-to-eat	¾ cup
Cornmeal (dry)	3 Tablespoons
Cream of Wheat or Rice Cereals (cooked)	½ cup
Flour (dry)	3 Tablespoons
Granola, low-fat	¼ cup
Grits	½ cup
Muesli	¼ cup

Oats (cooked)	½ cup
Pasta	1/3 cup
Puffed cereal	1.5 cups
Rice, white or brown	1/3 cup
Shredded Wheat	1/3 cup
Sugar-frosted cereal	½ cup

Beans, Peas, and Lentils: One Food Choice

Beans and peas (cooked) (garbanzo, pinto, kidney, white, split, black-eyed)	½ cup
Lima beans (cooked)	2/3 cup
Lentils (cooked)	½ cup

Starchy Vegetables: One Food Choice

Baked beans	1/3 cup
Corn	½ cup
Corn on the cob, medium	1 (5 oz)
Mixed vegetables with corn, peas, or pasta	1 cup
Peas, green	½ cup
Potato, baked or boiled	1 small (3 oz)
Potato, mashed	½ cup
Squash, winter (acorn, butternut)	1 cup
Yam, sweet potato, plain	½ cup

Vegetables: FREE (all you can eat)

Artichoke
Mixed vegetables (without pasta, peas, corn)
Artichoke hearts   Mushrooms
Asparagus   Okra
Beans (green, wax, Italian)   Onions

Bean sprouts

Beets

Broccoli

Brussels sprouts

Salad greens (lettuce, romaine, spinach)

Cabbage

Carrots

Cauliflower

Celery

Cucumber

Eggplant

Green onions or scallions

Tomato/vegetable juice

Greens (collard, kale, mustard, turnip)

Kohlrabi

Leeks

Zucchini

Vegetable Soup (made with FREE vegetables)

Pea pods

Peppers (all varieties)

Radishes

Sauerkraut

Spinach

Summer squash

Tomato

Tomatoes, canned

Tomato sauce

Turnips

Water chestnuts

Watercress

Starchy Foods Prepared with Fat: One Food Choice

Biscuit, 2.5 in across	1
Chow mein noodles	½ cup
Corn bread, 2 in cube	1 (2 oz)
Crackers, round butter type	6
Croutons	1 cup
French-fried potatoes	16-25 (3 oz)
Granola	¼ cup
Muffin, plain small	1 (1.5 oz)
Pancake, 4 in across	2
Popcorn, microwave	3 cups
Sandwich crackers, cheese or peanut filling	3
Stuffing, bread (prepared)	1/3 cup
Taco shell, 6 in square	2
Waffle, 4.5 in square	1
Whole-wheat crackers, fat added	4-6 (1 oz)

Crackers and Snacks: One Food Choice

Animal crackers	8
Graham crackers, 2.5 in square	3
Matzoh	¾ oz
Melba toast	4 slices
Oyster crackers	24
Popcorn (popped, no fat added or low-fat microwave)	3 cups
Pretzels	¾ oz
Rice cakes, 4 in across	2
Saltine-type crackers	6
Snack chips, fat-free (tortilla, potato)	15-20 (3/4 oz)
Whole-wheat crackers, no fat added	2-5 (3/4 oz)

Milk: One Food Choice

Skim milk	1 cup
½% milk	1 cup
1% milk	1 cup
Nonfat or low-fat buttermilk	1 cup
Evaporated skim milk	½ cup
Plain nonfat yogurt	¾ cup
2% milk	¾ cup
Plain low-fat yogurt	¾ cup
Whole milk	1 cup
Evaporated whole milk	½ cup

Fruit Juice: One Food Choice

Apple juice/cider	½ cup
Cranberry juice cocktail	1/3 cup
Cranberry juice cocktail, reduced-calorie	1 cup
Fruit juice blends, 100% juice	1/3 cup

Grape juice	1/3 cup
Grapefruit juice	½ cup
Orange juice	½ cup
Pineapple juice	½ cup
Prune juice	1/3 cup

Fruit: One Food Choice

Apple, unpeeled, small	1 (4 oz)
Applesauce, unsweetened	½ cup
Apples, dried	4 rings
Apricots, fresh	4 whole, (5.5 oz)
Apricots, dried	8 halves
Apricots, canned	½ cup
Banana, small	1 (4 oz)
Blackberries	¾ cup
Blueberries	¾ cup
Cantaloupe, small cubes	1/3 melon (11 oz) or 1 cup
Cherries, sweet, fresh	12 (3 oz)
Cherries, sweet, canned	½ cup
Dates	3
Figs, fresh	1.5 large or 2 medium (3.5 oz)
Figs, dried	1.5
Fruit cocktail	½ cup
Grapefruit, large	½ (11 oz)
Grapefruits sections, canned	¾ cup
Grapes, small	17 (3 oz)
Honeydew melon	1 slice (10 oz) or 1 cup cubes
Kiwi	1 (3.5 oz)
Mandarin oranges, canned	¾ cup
Mango, small	½ fruit (5.5 oz) or ½ cup
Nectarine, small	1 (5 oz)
Orange, small	1 (6.5 oz)
Papaya	½ fruit (8 oz) or 1 cup cubes
Peach, medium, fresh	1 (6 oz)
Peaches, canned	½ cup
Pear, large, fresh	½ (4 oz)

Pears, canned	½ cup
Pineapple, fresh	¾ cup
Pineapple, canned	½ cup
Plums, small	2 (5 oz)
Plums, canned	½ cup
Prunes, dried	3
Raisins	2 tablespoons
Raspberries	1 cup
Strawberries	1.25 cups whole berries
Tangerines, small	2 (8 oz)
Watermelon	1 slice (13.5 oz) or 1.25 cup cubes

Other Carbohydrates: One Food Choice

Angel food cake, unfrosted	1/24th of cake
Brownie, small, unfrosted	2 in square
Cake, unfrosted	1 in square
Chili with beans	½ cup
Cole Slaw	½ cup
Cookie, fat free	2 small
Cookie or sandwich cookie	2 small
Cranberry sauce, jellied	¼ cup
Cupcake, frosted	½ small
Doughnut, plain cake	2/3 medium
Doughnut, glazed (3.75 in across)	½ item
Fruit juice bars (100% juice)	1 (3 oz)
Fruit snacks, chewy	1 roll (3/4 oz)
Fruit spreads, 100% fruit)	1 tablespoon
Gelatin, regular	½ cup
Gingersnaps	3 cookies
Granola bar	1 bar
Honey	1 tablespoon
Ice Cream	½ cup
Ice Cream, light	½ cup
Ice Cream, fat free, no sugar	½ cup
Jam or jelly, regular	1 tablespoon
Macaroni salad	½ cup

Milk, chocolate, whole	½ cup
Pie, fruit, 2 crusts	1/18th
Pie, pumpkin or custard	1/16th
Potato chips	12-18 (1 oz)
Potato Salad	½ cup
Pudding with low-fat milk	¼ cup
Pudding, sugar free	½ cup
Salad dressing, fat-free	½ cup
Sherbet, sorbet	¼ cup
Spaghetti or pasta sauce	½ cup
Sugar	1 tablespoon
Sweet roll or Danish	1/3 roll
Syrup, light	2 tablespoons
Syrup, regular	1 tablespoon
Tortilla chips	6-12 (1 oz)
Vanilla Wafers	5 cookies
Vegetable soup (with potatoes, peas and corn)	1 cup
Yogurt frozen, low-fat, fat-free	1/3 cup
Yogurt, frozen, fat-free, no sugar	½ cup
Yogurt, low fat with fruit	1/3 cup

TROUBLESHOOTING GUIDE

The poet W. H. Auden famously said, "poetry makes nothing happen". Perhaps he was referring to weight loss. It is in this spirit that these additional poems are offered.

SUPPLEMENTAL POEMS

Support

Twenty-third Pound

"Our weight loss sermon for this Sunday comes from the King Carl version of The Poet's Weight Loss Plan"

These guidelines are my shepherd.
I shall not indulge.
They direct me to eat meat and vegetables;
they steer me from excessive portions.
They restore my proper weight,
through the careful avoidance of carbohydrates
and weekly fasting.
Yea, though I push my cart down the central aisles,
I will not purchase.
Though I am stopped in check out between all these impulse
bargains,
I will not buy.
They describe an effective diet strategy from among so many
pretenders,
and bleed me of my fat.
For - combined with *Intermittent Fasting* - the advice is
scientifically sound,
and will sustain my weight throughout the days of my life.

Tips

Crowd Sourcing / Snacks and Food That Comes in Crowds

Again and again,
they arrive like army ants
flooding through the carefully placed barricades
of your diet:
bite-sized food, finger food, snack food, prepared food, ready-to-eat
nibbles, cheezits, donut holes, chips of all sorts, cheese and crackers,
thingies on toothpicks, mouth-sized snacks, candies, popcorn, nuts,
cookies, chocolate kisses, bon bons (eat them quickly before they
melt!), jelly beans, etc.
All the work has been done.
 You just pop them into your mouth.
Or not.

We're here to talk about the "or not".
Basically, *don't eat anything which has been pre-made bite-sized.*
(You may let someone cut your food for you.)
Avoid whatever's quick.
You'll notice thin people do this.
Oh they just chop, chop, chop
and taste, taste, taste,
and stir, stir, stir...
Then never eat!
What is wrong with them?
(Personally, I need a glass of wine to watch it.)

But we can learn from them.
Anything that lengthens the path from possible food
to your mouth
is free dietary assistance, free discipline.

Do not outsource your intake.
Prepare and eat only large, whole things
like hams, chickens, tomatoes, lettuce heads, a side of beef...
Be like that ant carrying off that crumb ten times its size,
only make it a carrot.

Dogs

A person who watches their dog's weight
will tend to watch their own.
I don't know why.
But a dog who waddles about like a footstool is
depressing.
Perhaps we read too much of ourselves into our dogs.
Nevertheless, it can be put to use.
Place the dog on a strict diet.
Once your dog has become trim,
it will have an effect upon you.
I don't know why.

How does a dog fit into your diet?
However you want.
Dogs are like that.

Temptations

Eve's recollection

"Oh, but we didn't just eat the apple.
We cooked and fermented it
and woke up with mud
on the one side of our face
and stars on the other."

Soda Pop

The fact that you are reading this
means that you are in dire trouble.
Look at that moist can side for goodness sakes!
It's all sugar, some chemicals and
a portion of some town's aquifer.
There was absolutely no reason for you to purchase this.

Go drink several glasses of water
until this makes sense to you.
You are dehydrated.

Chocolate

The important thing is
to not show fear.
Chocolate can sense fear
in a dieting person,
especially women,
and insinuate itself
back into their good graces
by threatening to leave.

They will ask you to imagine a world
without them.
They ask,
"Is this what you really want?"
"Do you want to live in a world without chocolate?"

Eat it.
That will shut it up.
But just the one raising its voice.
Not all the others.

These Foods Which Run In Crowds

Cherries and grapes are tricky.
Not so many calories by themselves,
yet they run in bunches.
You get the idea.
These foods which run in crowds
sorely try the discipline.
Potato chip, or chips? Peanut, or peanuts?
There are so many lines being crossed
between levels of temptation -
how am I to earn a looser belt?

Potato Chips

Snack companies spend millions
employing all the knowledge of science
to entice you to eat that next chip.
And if that isn't enough,
they hand you the dip,
giving it the flavor latitude
of all the food groups
so that this potato chip
can be virtually
anything you would want it to be.
It's your taste buds' perfect world.
What's a sinner to do?

Ask yourself,
"Why did this potato chip cross the table?"
And the answer is:
because *you* are there.
Don't look.
Move away.

The Morning Danish, Almond Croissant or Bear Claw
add powdered sugar for an extra dusting of sin

Food doesn't get any faster than this.
They were ready to go
long before you were up
and out the door.
They even precede coffee
in many of the written histories.

Cake

"You can have your cake
and eat it too."
This is so true for dieters.
You will wear that cake for a long time.

Remember the last time someone
baked you a cake?
That's about how often
you should eat some.

Pasta
Saying 'Basta!' to pasta.

This is a tough one.
Who doesn't like the Italians,
even their Godfather?
But they and their sauces can get heavy.
Don't get in wrong with these people,
as they say.

Bagels with Cream Cheese

Flour based breads and pastas
with their quick release carbohydrates
could yet up-end civilization.

Your fingers should burn
when touching white flour.
The fragrance of fresh bread
should sting your nose.

Baring this,
try to eat them with some
egg or protein.
And as for the next time,

"Horseman, pass by."

Gravies and Sauces

"One bite can make you larger,…"

need to be addressed.
A diet is not the high life.
Rich foods build poor people.

The Road to Hell
was built with Good Intentions
and fueled by Rich Foods.

Gravies and sauces
dribble in and about
regular portions
crossing the borders of scrupulous caloric calculation
with seeming impunity
yet still accounting for a sizeable percentage
of the Gross Caloric Intake, or GCI.

Common Questions & Feelings

Reaching the Horse Latitudes at the Forty-fifth Pound

We've been stalled at the forty-fifth pound parallel
for several months, and restive
staring at an unmoving horizon
on a vast mirroring sea of patent resolve,

tossing edibles overboard
in an effort to lighten,
sipping from a thimble, it would seem,
and eating salted eggs.
And now the Captain orders
that when we reach our goal,
what we eat then will remain so.
Oh!

We passed a set point not far back
where perhaps we should have stopped
to refresh and replenish.
The natives there still have some flesh on them.
I could grow used to a little paunch
around the bow.

It's not so bad, and
I'd never thought of flab in quite this way,
but it feels a lot like relaxation,
maybe even like liberation.
More flesh, maybe, is needed.

Haunted

I am haunted by the ever-present,
all-to-evident, bubble wrap of me
taking over as my fat index climbs.

It's a great burden I carry,
trudging up the hill with
my twin.
It's an exorcism, I need.

So many nutritionists have muttered,
recipes, counted calories, assigned "Hail Marys"
(exercise regimens)
and chastised my mother,
and her mother
as Depression Era deplorables
of the lard based times...
I'm told I need to separate her
from these sins.
"Love the sinner, hate the sin."

Can't I love them *both*?
Isn't love all there is?
Please?

Twenty-sixth Pound
Channeling My Fat

You have never embraced me!
 I have always been second-class flesh.
You never compliment me.
How many times have I wanted just one more glazed donut
and you've said, "No"?
You have done everything short of surgical intervention
to make me disappear.
You purposely pace activities
which you *know*
it will be hard for me to maintain!
Why do you hate me so?
All I've ever done is to give of myself.

Slender

They may be greasy, scrawny weasels,
who'd steal from their mothers
and rob dead people,
abuse their wives, smoke, drink
and sport garish tattoos
on their pipe stem arms...
All the same, they're slender,
and you envy them.

Mealtime

Oh, happy hour!
My good fortune floweth over.
I relish dining, snacking, chewing, sipping, tasting,
nibbling, sniffing and sipping.
I have a nudist's carefree abandon with it all.

If it dribbles down my chin,
or glosses my lips,
or decorates my nose,
or obscures my vision...
I'm one with it all!
Sure, the whole buffet.
Bring it on!

Fried food, dipped food, BBQ'd, caramelized,
baked or boiled, processed or reduced,
wild or farmed,
foreign or domestic,
carbonated or fizzle free,
popular or fringe-fare,
fast or slow,
spicy or mild,
hot or cold,
with everything or plain,
sugar enhanced or chocolate covered,
everything but the barely killed
- I'm good with.

I really hate to see it twitch.

Fasting is Like Grieving

First of all there's the absence,
which is total.
Second is the presence;
memories everywhere you look.
Shadows walking about
without their maker.
They pass between walls;
they pass between rooms.
Odors are everywhere,
when I'm not eating.

Like my father-in-law who is gone,
I spend more of my time thinking about him.
As if he could use the help now,
staying substantial.

ADDENDUM: THE FAST TRACK

Maintaining discipline often demands a settled structure. A comfortable discipline leans on the accumulation of habit. We exercise regularly. We eat regular meals regularly. We do our regular activities. We can leave a lot of these activities to the habitual autopilot. But when our lives are tossed into disarray or altered greatly, our habitual autopilot switches off and we are back into minute by minute control. As we've discussed above, in these cases our reserves of discipline are depleted rapidly.

The Covid-19 pandemic was such a disturbance for me. Our son returned home. He is a great cook. Our schedule became erratic. Instead of two meals and a snack, I began eating three. The meals were tastier, with bigger portions and with more carbohydrates - such as my son preferred. I still fasted one day/week, but over a period of three months I ballooned twenty pounds.

When our son left for a job out of town, I decided it was time to resume my dietary discipline. But instead of fasting one day/week and eating the correct portions by the book, I decided I would like to try losing the extra pounds at a faster rate. I have begun to fast every other day. Indeed, fasting correctly is easier than eating correctly. And I've found that I haven't had any real difficulty in fasting every other day, when I can look forward to breaking the fast every other day. The fasting is easier in some respects, because I experience the fat being lost faster. This sense of speed is helpful.

So, I would recommend this schedule for a faster weight loss. But I would recommend using fasting one day/week as per the initial discipline for beginners, until they have lost thirty or so pounds over a six month or so period. Fasting and eating properly are skills that require practice.

If you do elect to try the Fast Track to weight loss, I would caution you to take your electrolyte pills on the days you fast. Fainting is most apt to occur the morning after, when you resume eating. Taking your electrolyte pills will ameliorate this. Also eating a small portion, then waiting an half hour to eat another small portion, and waiting to eat your regular portions for a couple hours or so can prevent those great shifts of fluid volumes from the blood into the intestines which I believe are responsible for the faints and lightheadedness. As in most things, prudence and moderation are best.

ABOUT THE AUTHOR

Carl Nelson received his MD from the University of Washington in 1975, but has never practiced. Instead he followed his Muse into painting, writing, the theater and poetry. There is probably no professional who understands failure as well as those in the arts, nor who must search so assiduously for the means and will to persist not only in their profession but in life itself. To do so, the author has held a number of part-time employments, many of which have as their sole requisite being the ability to endure e.g. telemarketer, bus driver, warehouse worker, laborer. In continuing to produce his art, Carl Nelson believes he has developed certain strategies with which to enhance and augment the will to persist through both numbing routine and deflating encounters which has brought some perspective to this book.

He has used his experiences in creating *The Poet's Weight Loss Plan* with which he has achieved his personal goal of a currently sustained weight loss of 40 pounds.

He is presently thriving in Belpre, Ohio with his wife, son and a ginger dachshund named Tater Tot, with whom he moseys about. He currently writes poems and essays which have been published in numerous journals. He also runs the Serenity Poetry Series in Marietta, Ohio. Find out more about Carl and his books at: amazon.com/author/nelsoncarl

[i] "100 Million Dieters, $20 Billion: The Weight-Loss Industry by the Numbers," ABC News online, last modified May 8, 2012. http://abcnews.go.com/Health/100-million-dieters-20-billion-weight-loss-industry/story?id=16297197.

[ii] "Diet starts today... and ends on Friday: How we quickly slip back into bad eating habits within a few days," *Daily Mail* online, last modified September 16, 2013. http://www.dailymail.co.uk/news/article-2421737/Diet-starts-today--ends-Friday-How-quickly-slip-bad-eating-habits-days.html. The snapshot of the nation's dieting habits has been revealed in a survey of more than 2,000 Britons by Alpro, a company advocating plant-based eating.

[iii] Sass, Cynthia. "5 Reasons Most Diets Fail Within 7 Days," *Health* online, last modified September 19, 2003. http://www.health.com/nutrition/5-reasons-most-diets-fail-within-7-days.

[iv] Monastyrsky, Konstantin. "The Real Reason Diets Fail and What You Can Do About It," The Health Home Economist, last modified January 25, 2018. http://www.thehealthyhomeeconomist.com/the-real-reason-diets-fail-and-what-you-can-do-about-it/.

[v] Ibid.

[vi] "Set-Point Theory," Center for Health Promotion & Wellness at MIT Medical, September 20, 2006, https://medical.mit.edu/sites/default/files/set_point_theory.pdf. Adapted from *Integrative Group Treatment for Bulimia Nervosa* by Helen Riess, M.D. and Mary Dockray-Miller.

[vii] "Is It a Myth That Muscle Burns More Calories Than Fat?"Livestrong.com, last accessed 28 June 2018. http://www.livestrong.com/article/447243-is-it-a-myth-that-muscle-burns-more-calories-than-fat/

[viii] "Understanding Metabolism: What Determines Your BMR?" FitDay, last accessed 23 June 2018. https://www.fitday.com/fitness-articles/nutrition/understanding-metabolism-what-determines-your-bmr.html.

www.ingramcontent.com/pod-product-compliance
Lightning Source LLC
Chambersburg PA
CBHW072131280526

45788CB00002B/592